The Relaxation Solution

Workbook and Journal

By Stephen Diamond

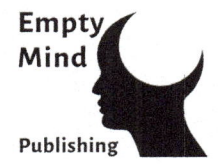

Empty Mind Publishing

Copyright © 2022 by Stephen Diamond
Cover art © by Alina Osadchenko, licensed by Dreamstime.
Cover design by Stephen Diamond

Published by Empty Mind Publishing LLC
Tucson, AZ 85748
emptymindpublishing.com

All rights reserved. No part of this publication may be reproduced, distributed, or transmitted in any form or by any means, including photocopying, recording, or other electronic or mechanical methods, without the prior written permission of the publisher, except in the case of brief quotations embodied in book reviews and certain other noncommercial uses permitted by copyright law.

This book details the author's personal experiences with and opinions about stress relief. The author is not your healthcare provider, and this book is not intended as a substitute for the medical advice of psychologists or physicians. Individual results vary. You should consult a physician in matters relating to your health and particularly with respect to any symptoms that may require diagnosis or medical attention.

ISBN 979-8-9862949-5-7

Praise for *The Relaxation Solution*

If you want temporary relief from worldly tension, take a hot bath. If you want permanent mindful relief, read this book, do the exercises and thank Stephen Diamond.

-Rolland Smith, poet, correspondent, and 11-time Emmy Award-winning television journalist

---

This is my favorite mindfulness book. It's written with a light touch, and we can feel Steve's generosity and good cheer shine from every page. What I find most exciting is Steve's new approach. He introduces us to a mindfulness that's naturally open, easygoing and relaxing. And what I find most impressive is the chapter on Awareness, which builds on the self-help perspective and invites us to discover an infinite source of spaciousness, relaxation and freedom from stress.

Greg Goode, author of *Standing As Awareness, The Direct Path, After Awareness*; editor of *Real-World Nonduality: Reports from the Field*

The Relaxation Solution is written from the standpoint of a caring friend. From body to mind to awareness to love, Stephen clears the cobwebs of false expectations and takes us on a practiced journey into awareness and release of unwanted tension. Engaging and practical for everyday life.

Terry Stevens, author, singer, stroke survivor, multi-exhibited fine artist

Table of Contents

Praise for *The Relaxation Solution* — 3
Epigraph — 5
Introduction — 6
How to Use This Book — 7
Workbook and Journal Pages — 10
Was This Book Helpful? — 441
About the Author — 442

Epigraph

It's very important that we re-learn the art of resting and relaxing. Not only does it help prevent the onset of many illnesses that develop through chronic tension and worrying; it allows us to clear our minds, focus, and find creative solutions to problems.
—Thích Nhất Hạnh

The Relaxation Solution Workbook and Journal

Introduction

Stress is literally killing us. I only wish I were exaggerating. Sorry to say, the science backs it up 100%. Multiple studies over the years have shown that stress from a variety of causes—social isolation, depression, unemployment, anxiety attacks, to name a few—can alter our bodies at the cellular level, potentially causing chronic diseases and even premature death.

In this modern age we are surrounded with things that cause us stress. Our jobs, our finances, our relationships, the environment, war, politics, news, advertising, social media. It can feel like we're constantly bombarded with stressful situations. They're almost impossible to avoid.

How we respond to these stressors makes all the difference. Do we let them get to us? Or can we remain calm in the midst of the storm?

This workbook will help you keep track of how you're responding to the stressors in your life. It will help you become aware of your patterns and habits. Once you're aware, you'll be able to change. Without that awareness, change is impossible.

For much more on this topic, see my book *The Relaxation Solution: The Secret to Stress-Free Living*. It's likely to be available wherever you bought this workbook. Or you can request it from your local bookstore or public library.

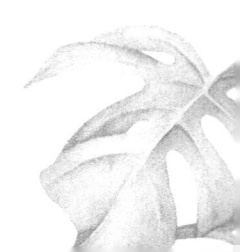

The Relaxation Solution Workbook and Journal

How to Use This Book

This is the companion to my book, *The Relaxation Solution*, which I hope you'll consider acquiring. You can use this workbook on its own. I'll tell you how. But you'll really get more out of it if you read the explanations behind the exercises and, above all, do the specific exercises I recommend. With *The Relaxation Solution* you get exclusive online access to 35 minutes of audios recorded by me, which you can stream or download, that take you through each exercise step by step.

This workbook has three types of pages: Daily Journal, Weekly Check-In, Monthly (4-week) Self-Evaluation. Here's how to use them.

Daily Journal

You'll devote most of your attention to these pages. The book contains a full year's worth (52 weeks, 364 days). I've deliberately not boxed in the columns on each line. If you have leftover lines, feel free to write free-form notes.

Theme of the Day

> This may come to mind at the beginning or end of the day, or anytime in between. There's no need to force it. If no theme occurs to you some days, leave this blank or make a doodle!

Exercises I Did

> List the exercises and meditations you did today. You can follow the program from *The Relaxation Solution* book or any other meditation program that appeals to you. If they're ones from *The Relaxation Solution*, you may want to note the exercise number here. Use the *notes* column to remind yourself of anything special that happened or of the general feeling.

The Relaxation Solution Workbook and Journal

Tension I Observed

> List instances when you noticed specific tensions during the day. If there was a triggering event and an emotion associated with the tension, jot it down. Be specific about where in the body you felt the tension and about what resolution came about, if any. Did you find the effort you were making to sustain the tension? Did you let it go?

Relaxation Remembrance

> List the attention-getting devices and reminders you're using (see *The Relaxation Solution*, chapter six) to help you remember to look for tension and let it go. Circle Y or N according to whether the reminder is still working. If not, find something new for tomorrow.

Mood Check

> This is for fun, and it's also an important cumulative record of how you're doing. Mark the emoji that most closely resembles your mood!

Weekly Check-In

Theme of the Week

> If it seems to you that the week has had a theme, write it here. If not, leave this blank or make a doodle!

Notes to Self

> This is your space to write whatever comes up. It's free-form journaling. Enjoy it!

Monthly Self-Evaluation

One of these is at the start of the book, and then every four weeks thereafter. There are 14 altogether. Since the book is organized in 4-week intervals rather than calendar months, you

The Relaxation Solution Workbook and Journal

can begin to use it any time. As you continue to practice the exercises, you can expect your stress levels to improve.

This questionnaire is based on the Perceived Stress Scale (PSS), as originally developed in 1983 by Cohen, Kamarck and Mermelstein. PSS is widely used as a self-reporting tool for stress management.

You'll find detailed instructions and scoring on each Self-Evaluation page. Just remember that it's important to answer honestly. This is for you, not for anyone else.

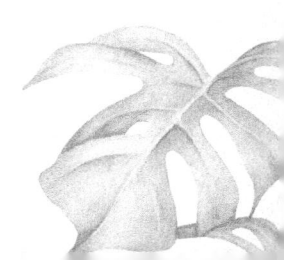

The Relaxation Solution Workbook and Journal

Workbook and Journal Pages

Tension is a habit. Relaxing is a habit. Bad habits can be broken, good habits formed.
—William James

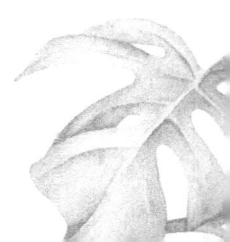

The Relaxation Solution

Monthly Self-Evaluation

Today is _____

M T W T F S S

Instructions

Thinking about your life during the past month, answer each question honestly. Don't try to add up specific events. Just respond with your impression or estimate. Write your answer in the *raw* column.

Answers

0 – never   1 – rarely   2 – sometimes   3 – often   4 – very often

Questions

answer: raw   adj

1. How often have you been upset because of something that happened unexpectedly? ___ → ___

2. How often have you felt that you were unable to control the important things in your life? ___ → ___

3. How often have you felt nervous and stressed? ___ → ___

4. How often have you felt confident about your ability to handle your personal problems? ___ 4↘ ___

5. How often have you felt that things were going your way? ___ 4↘ ___

6. How often have you found that you could not cope with all the things that you had to do? ___ → ___

7. How often have you been able to control irritations in your life? ___ 4↘ ___

8. How often have you felt that you were on top of things? ___ 4↘ ___

9. How often have you been angered because of things that happened outside of your control? ___ → ___

10. How often have you felt difficulties were piling up so high you could not overcome them? ___ → ___

Total: ___

Scoring

Write an adjusted score in the *adj* column. To calculate *adj*:
For questions 4, 5, 7, and 8, subtract raw score from 4
(change 0 to 4, 1 to 3, 2 to 2, 3 to 1, and 4 to 0.)
For questions 1, 2, 3, 6, 9, and 10, copy the raw score into *adj*.

Evaluation

If your total adjusted score is...

0 to 13 - your stress level is **low**.
14 to 26 - your stress level is **moderate**.
27 to 40 - your stress level is **high**.

The Relaxation Solution
Daily Journal

Today is _____

M T W T F S S

Theme of the Day

Exercises I Did
time — *duration* — *exercise* — *notes*

Tension I Observed
trigger — *emotion* — *body locations* — *resolution*

Relaxation Remembrance
trigger (sticker, red light...) — *working?*

Y N
Y N
Y N
Y N

Mood Check
morning

afternoon

evening

The Relaxation Solution
Daily Journal

Today is _____
M T W T F S S

Theme of the Day

Exercises I Did
time — *duration* — *exercise* — *notes*

Tension I Observed
trigger — *emotion* — *body locations* — *resolution*

Relaxation Remembrance
trigger (sticker, red light...) — *working?*

Y   N
Y   N
Y   N
Y   N

Mood Check
morning

afternoon

evening

The Relaxation Solution
Daily Journal

Today is _____
M T W T F S S

Theme of the Day

Exercises I Did
time — duration — exercise — notes

Tension I Observed
trigger — emotion — body locations — resolution

Relaxation Remembrance
trigger (sticker, red light...) — working?

Y N
Y N
Y N
Y N

Mood Check
morning

afternoon

evening

The Relaxation Solution
Daily Journal

Today is _____

M T W T F S S

Theme of the Day

Exercises I Did
time — duration — exercise — notes

Tension I Observed
trigger — emotion — body locations — resolution

Relaxation Remembrance
trigger (sticker, red light...) — working?

Y N
Y N
Y N
Y N

Mood Check
morning

afternoon

evening

The Relaxation Solution
Daily Journal

Today is _____

M T W T F S S

Theme of the Day

Exercises I Did
time — *duration* — *exercise* — *notes*

Tension I Observed
trigger — *emotion* — *body locations* — *resolution*

Relaxation Remembrance
trigger (sticker, red light...) — *working?*

Y N
Y N
Y N
Y N

Mood Check
morning

afternoon

evening

The Relaxation Solution
Daily Journal

Today is _____
M T W T F S S

Theme of the Day

Exercises I Did
time — *duration* — *exercise* — *notes*

Tension I Observed
trigger — *emotion* — *body locations* — *resolution*

Relaxation Remembrance
trigger (sticker, red light...) — *working?*

Y N
Y N
Y N
Y N

Mood Check
morning

afternoon

evening

The Relaxation Solution
Daily Journal

Today is _____

M T W T F S S

Theme of the Day

Exercises I Did
time — duration — exercise — notes

Tension I Observed
trigger — emotion — body locations — resolution

Relaxation Remembrance
trigger (sticker, red light...) — working?

- Y N
- Y N
- Y N
- Y N

Mood Check

morning

afternoon

evening

The Relaxation Solution
Weekly Journal

Today is _____
M T W T F S S

Theme of the Week

Notes to Self

The Relaxation Solution
Daily Journal

Today is _____

M T W T F S S

Theme of the Day

Exercises I Did
time — *duration* — *exercise* — *notes*

Tension I Observed
trigger — *emotion* — *body locations* — *resolution*

Relaxation Remembrance
trigger (sticker, red light...) — *working?*

Y N
Y N
Y N
Y N

Mood Check
morning

afternoon

evening

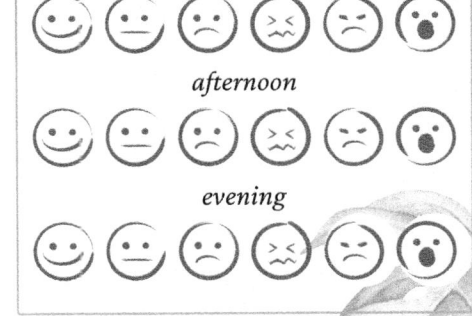

The Relaxation Solution
Daily Journal

Today is _____

M T W T F S S

Theme of the Day

Exercises I Did
time — *duration* — *exercise* — *notes*

Tension I Observed
trigger — *emotion* — *body locations* — *resolution*

Relaxation Remembrance
trigger (sticker, red light...) — *working?*

Y N
Y N
Y N
Y N

Mood Check

morning

afternoon

evening

The Relaxation Solution
Daily Journal

Today is _____

M T W T F S S

Theme of the Day

Exercises I Did
time — *duration* — *exercise* — *notes*

Tension I Observed
trigger — *emotion* — *body locations* — *resolution*

Relaxation Remembrance
trigger (sticker, red light...) — *working?*

- Y N
- Y N
- Y N
- Y N

Mood Check

morning

afternoon

evening

The Relaxation Solution
Daily Journal

Today is _____
M T W T F S S

Theme of the Day

Exercises I Did
time — duration — exercise — notes

Tension I Observed
trigger — emotion — body locations — resolution

Relaxation Remembrance
trigger (sticker, red light…) — *working?*

Y N
Y N
Y N
Y N

Mood Check
morning
afternoon
evening

The Relaxation Solution

Daily Journal

Today is _____

M T W T F S S

Theme of the Day

Exercises I Did

time — duration — exercise — notes

Tension I Observed

trigger — emotion — body locations — resolution

Relaxation Remembrance

trigger (sticker, red light...) — working?

Y N
Y N
Y N
Y N

Mood Check

morning

afternoon

evening

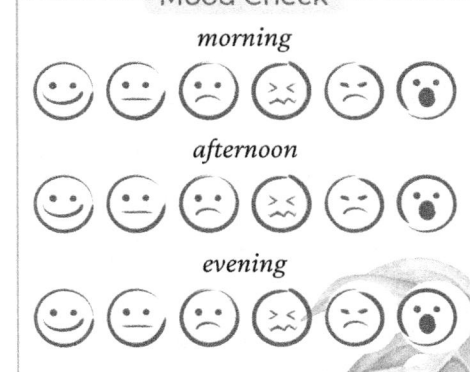

The Relaxation Solution
Daily Journal

Today is _____

M T W T F S S

Theme of the Day

Exercises I Did
time — *duration* — *exercise* — *notes*

Tension I Observed
trigger — *emotion* — *body locations* — *resolution*

Relaxation Remembrance
trigger (sticker, red light...) — *working?*

Y N
Y N
Y N
Y N

Mood Check
morning

afternoon

evening

The Relaxation Solution
Daily Journal

Today is _____
M T W T F S S

Theme of the Day

Exercises I Did
time — *duration* — *exercise* — *notes*

Tension I Observed
trigger — *emotion* — *body locations* — *resolution*

Relaxation Remembrance
trigger (sticker, red light...) — *working?*

- Y   N
- Y   N
- Y   N
- Y   N

Mood Check
morning

afternoon

evening

The Relaxation Solution

Weekly Journal

Today is _____

M T W T F S S

Theme of the Week

Notes to Self

The Relaxation Solution
Daily Journal

Today is _____

M T W T F S S

Theme of the Day

Exercises I Did
time — duration — exercise — notes

Tension I Observed
trigger — emotion — body locations — resolution

Relaxation Remembrance
trigger (sticker, red light...) — *working?*

Y N
Y N
Y N
Y N

Mood Check
morning
😊 😐 🙁 😣 😖 😮

afternoon
😊 😐 🙁 😣 😖 😮

evening
😊 😐 🙁 😣 😖 😮

The Relaxation Solution
Daily Journal

Today is _____
M T W T F S S

Theme of the Day

Exercises I Did
time — *duration* — *exercise* — *notes*

Tension I Observed
trigger — *emotion* — *body locations* — *resolution*

Relaxation Remembrance
trigger (sticker, red light...) — *working?*

Y N
Y N
Y N
Y N

Mood Check
morning
afternoon
evening

The Relaxation Solution
Daily Journal

Today is _____

M T W T F S S

Theme of the Day

Exercises I Did
time — *duration* — *exercise* — *notes*

Tension I Observed
trigger — *emotion* — *body locations* — *resolution*

Relaxation Remembrance
trigger (sticker, red light...) — *working?*

Y N
Y N
Y N
Y N

Mood Check
morning

afternoon

evening

The Relaxation Solution
Daily Journal

Today is _____
M T W T F S S

Theme of the Day

Exercises I Did
time — duration — exercise — notes

Tension I Observed
trigger — emotion — body locations — resolution

Relaxation Remembrance
trigger (sticker, red light...) — *working?*

Y N
Y N
Y N
Y N

Mood Check
morning

afternoon

evening

The Relaxation Solution
Daily Journal

Today is _____

M T W T F S S

Theme of the Day

Exercises I Did
time — duration — exercise — notes

Tension I Observed
trigger — emotion — body locations — resolution

Relaxation Remembrance
trigger (sticker, red light...) — working?

Y N
Y N
Y N
Y N

Mood Check
morning

afternoon

evening

The Relaxation Solution
Daily Journal

Today is _____
M T W T F S S

Theme of the Day

Exercises I Did
time — *duration* — *exercise* — *notes*

Tension I Observed
trigger — *emotion* — *body locations* — *resolution*

Relaxation Remembrance
trigger (sticker, red light...) — *working?*

Y N
Y N
Y N
Y N

Mood Check
morning

afternoon

evening

The Relaxation Solution
Daily Journal

Today is _____
M T W T F S S

Theme of the Day

Exercises I Did
time — *duration* — *exercise* — *notes*

Tension I Observed
trigger — *emotion* — *body locations* — *resolution*

Relaxation Remembrance
trigger (sticker, red light...) — *working?*

Y N
Y N
Y N
Y N

Mood Check
morning

afternoon

evening

The Relaxation Solution

Weekly Journal

Today is _____

M T W T F S S

Theme of the Week

Notes to Self

The Relaxation Solution
Daily Journal

Today is _____

M T W T F S S

Theme of the Day

Exercises I Did
time	duration	exercise	notes

Tension I Observed
trigger	emotion	body locations	resolution

Relaxation Remembrance
trigger (sticker, red light...) — working?

- _____ Y N
- _____ Y N
- _____ Y N
- _____ Y N

Mood Check
morning

afternoon

evening

The Relaxation Solution
Daily Journal

Today is _____
M T W T F S S

Theme of the Day

Exercises I Did
time — *duration* — *exercise* — *notes*

Tension I Observed
trigger — *emotion* — *body locations* — *resolution*

Relaxation Remembrance
trigger (sticker, red light...) — *working?*

Y N
Y N
Y N
Y N

Mood Check
morning

afternoon

evening

The Relaxation Solution
Daily Journal

Today is _____

M T W T F S S

Theme of the Day

Exercises I Did
time — duration — exercise — notes

Tension I Observed
trigger — emotion — body locations — resolution

Relaxation Remembrance
trigger (sticker, red light...) — working?

Y N
Y N
Y N
Y N

Mood Check
morning

afternoon

evening

The Relaxation Solution
Daily Journal

Today is _____

M T W T F S S

Theme of the Day

Exercises I Did
time — *duration* — *exercise* — *notes*

Tension I Observed
trigger — *emotion* — *body locations* — *resolution*

Relaxation Remembrance
trigger (sticker, red light...) — *working?*

Y N
Y N
Y N
Y N

Mood Check
morning

afternoon

evening

The Relaxation Solution
Daily Journal

Today is _____

M   T   W   T   F   S   S

Theme of the Day

Exercises I Did
time — duration — exercise — notes

Tension I Observed
trigger — emotion — body locations — resolution

Relaxation Remembrance
trigger (sticker, red light...) — working?

Y   N
Y   N
Y   N
Y   N

Mood Check
morning

afternoon

evening

The Relaxation Solution
Daily Journal

Today is _____

M T W T F S S

Theme of the Day

Exercises I Did

time — *duration* — *exercise* — *notes*

Tension I Observed

trigger — *emotion* — *body locations* — *resolution*

Relaxation Remembrance

trigger (sticker, red light...) — *working?*

Y N
Y N
Y N
Y N

Mood Check

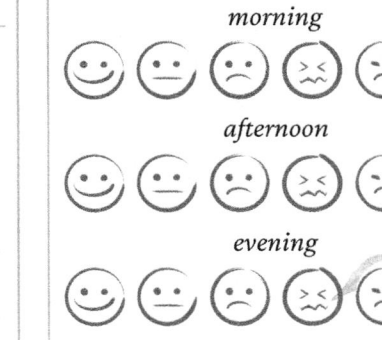

morning

afternoon

evening

The Relaxation Solution
Daily Journal

Today is _____

M T W T F S S

Theme of the Day

Exercises I Did
time — *duration* — *exercise* — *notes*

Tension I Observed
trigger — *emotion* — *body locations* — *resolution*

Relaxation Remembrance
trigger (sticker, red light...) — *working?*

Y N
Y N
Y N
Y N

Mood Check
morning

afternoon

evening

The Relaxation Solution

Weekly Journal

Today is _____

M T W T F S S

Theme of the Week

Notes to Self

The Relaxation Solution
Monthly Self-Evaluation

Today is _____

M T W T F S S

Instructions

Thinking about your life during the past month, answer each question honestly. Don't try to add up specific events. Just respond with your impression or estimate. Write your answer in the *raw* column.

Answers

0 – never   1 – rarely   2 – sometimes   3 – often   4 – very often

Questions

answer: — raw — adj

1. How often have you been upset because of something that happened unexpectedly? → ___
2. How often have you felt that you were unable to control the important things in your life? → ___
3. How often have you felt nervous and stressed? → ___
4. How often have you felt confident about your ability to handle your personal problems? 4-↘ ___
5. How often have you felt that things were going your way? 4-↘ ___
6. How often have you found that you could not cope with all the things that you had to do? → ___
7. How often have you been able to control irritations in your life? 4-↘ ___
8. How often have you felt that you were on top of things? 4-↘ ___
9. How often have you been angered because of things that happened outside of your control? → ___
10. How often have you felt difficulties were piling up so high you could not overcome them? → ___

Total: ___

Scoring

Write an adjusted score in the *adj* column. To calculate *adj*:
For questions 4, 5, 7, and 8, subtract raw score from 4
(change 0 to 4, 1 to 3, 2 to 2, 3 to 1, and 4 to 0.)
For questions 1, 2, 3, 6, 9, and 10, copy the raw score into *adj*.

Evaluation

If your total adjusted score is…

0 to 13 - your stress level is **low**.
14 to 26 - your stress level is **moderate**.
27 to 40 - your stress level is **high**.

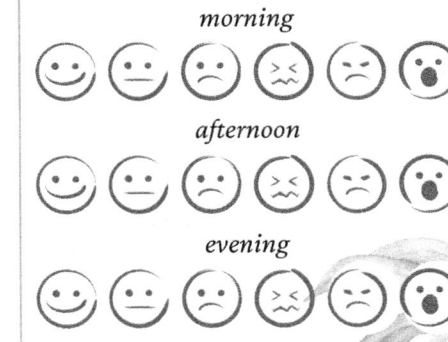

The Relaxation Solution
Daily Journal

Today is _____
M T W T F S S

Theme of the Day

Exercises I Did
time — *duration* — *exercise* — *notes*

Tension I Observed
trigger — *emotion* — *body locations* — *resolution*

Relaxation Remembrance
trigger (sticker, red light...) — *working?*

Y   N
Y   N
Y   N
Y   N

Mood Check
morning

afternoon

evening

The Relaxation Solution
Daily Journal

Today is _____

M T W T F S S

Theme of the Day

Exercises I Did
time — *duration* — *exercise* — *notes*

Tension I Observed
trigger — *emotion* — *body locations* — *resolution*

Relaxation Remembrance
trigger (sticker, red light...) — working?

- Y N
- Y N
- Y N
- Y N

Mood Check
morning

afternoon

evening

The Relaxation Solution
Daily Journal

Today is _____
M T W T F S S

Theme of the Day

Exercises I Did
time — duration — exercise — notes

Tension I Observed
trigger — emotion — body locations — resolution

Relaxation Remembrance
trigger (sticker, red light...) — working?

- Y N
- Y N
- Y N
- Y N

Mood Check
morning

afternoon

evening

The Relaxation Solution
Daily Journal

Today is _____

M T W T F S S

Theme of the Day

Exercises I Did

time — *duration* — *exercise* — *notes*

Tension I Observed

trigger — *emotion* — *body locations* — *resolution*

Relaxation Remembrance

trigger (sticker, red light...) — *working?*

Y   N

Y   N

Y   N

Y   N

Mood Check

morning

afternoon

evening

The Relaxation Solution
Daily Journal

Today is _____
M T W T F S S

Theme of the Day

Exercises I Did
time — *duration* — *exercise* — *notes*

Tension I Observed
trigger — *emotion* — *body locations* — *resolution*

Relaxation Remembrance
trigger (sticker, red light...) — *working?*

Y N
Y N
Y N
Y N

Mood Check
morning

afternoon

evening

The Relaxation Solution
Daily Journal

Today is _____
M T W T F S S

Theme of the Day

Exercises I Did
time — duration — exercise — notes

Tension I Observed
trigger — emotion — body locations — resolution

Relaxation Remembrance
trigger (sticker, red light...) — working?

Y   N
Y   N
Y   N
Y   N

Mood Check
morning

afternoon

evening

The Relaxation Solution
Daily Journal

Today is _____
M T W T F S S

Theme of the Day

Exercises I Did
time — duration — exercise — notes

Tension I Observed
trigger — emotion — body locations — resolution

Relaxation Remembrance
trigger (sticker, red light...) — working?

Y N
Y N
Y N
Y N

Mood Check
morning
afternoon
evening

The Relaxation Solution

Weekly Journal

Today is _____

M T W T F S S

--- Theme of the Week ---

--- Notes to Self ---

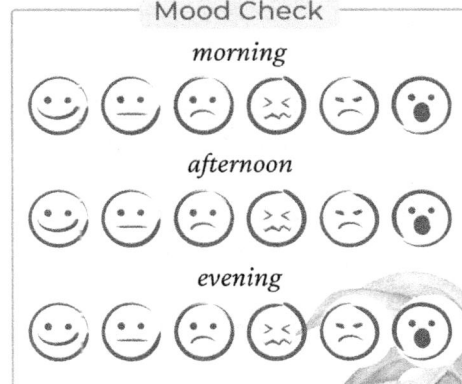

The Relaxation Solution
Daily Journal

Today is _____
M T W T F S S

Theme of the Day

Exercises I Did
time — *duration* — *exercise* — *notes*

Tension I Observed
trigger — *emotion* — *body locations* — *resolution*

Relaxation Remembrance
trigger (sticker, red light...) — *working?*

Y N
Y N
Y N
Y N

Mood Check
morning

afternoon

evening

The Relaxation Solution
Daily Journal

Today is _____
M T W T F S S

Theme of the Day

Exercises I Did
time — duration — exercise — notes

Tension I Observed
trigger — emotion — body locations — resolution

Relaxation Remembrance
trigger (sticker, red light…) — working?

Y N
Y N
Y N
Y N

Mood Check
morning

afternoon

evening

The Relaxation Solution
Daily Journal

Today is _____
M T W T F S S

Theme of the Day

Exercises I Did
— time — duration — exercise — notes —

Tension I Observed
— trigger — emotion — body locations — resolution —

Relaxation Remembrance
— trigger (sticker, red light…) — working? —

Y N
Y N
Y N
Y N

Mood Check
morning

afternoon

evening

The Relaxation Solution
Daily Journal

Today is _____
M T W T F S S

Theme of the Day

Exercises I Did
time — duration — exercise — notes

Tension I Observed
trigger — emotion — body locations — resolution

Relaxation Remembrance
trigger (sticker, red light...) — working?

- Y N
- Y N
- Y N
- Y N

Mood Check
morning

afternoon

evening

The Relaxation Solution
Daily Journal

Today is _____
M T W T F S S

Theme of the Day

Exercises I Did
time — *duration* — *exercise* — *notes*

Tension I Observed
trigger — *emotion* — *body locations* — *resolution*

Relaxation Remembrance
trigger (sticker, red light...) — *working?*

Y N
Y N
Y N
Y N

Mood Check
morning

afternoon

evening

The Relaxation Solution
Daily Journal

Today is _____
M T W T F S S

Theme of the Day

Exercises I Did
time — *duration* — *exercise* — *notes*

Tension I Observed
trigger — *emotion* — *body locations* — *resolution*

Relaxation Remembrance
trigger (sticker, red light...) — *working?*

Y   N
Y   N
Y   N
Y   N

Mood Check
morning
afternoon
evening

The Relaxation Solution
Daily Journal

Today is _____

M T W T F S S

Theme of the Day

Exercises I Did

time — *duration* — *exercise* — *notes*

Tension I Observed

trigger — *emotion* — *body locations* — *resolution*

Relaxation Remembrance

trigger (sticker, red light...) — *working?*

Y N
Y N
Y N
Y N

Mood Check

morning

afternoon

evening

The Relaxation Solution

Weekly Journal

Today is _____

M T W T F S S

Theme of the Week

Notes to Self

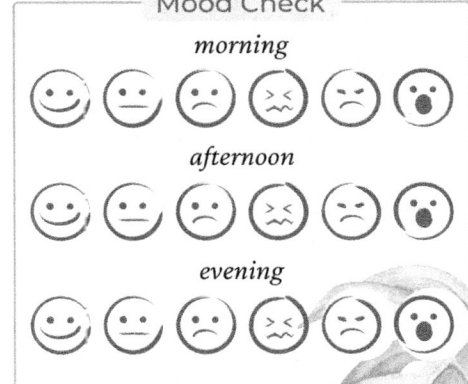

The Relaxation Solution
Daily Journal

Today is _____
M T W T F S S

Theme of the Day

Exercises I Did
time — *duration* — *exercise* — *notes*

Tension I Observed
trigger — *emotion* — *body locations* — *resolution*

Relaxation Remembrance
trigger (sticker, red light...) — *working?*

Y   N
Y   N
Y   N
Y   N

Mood Check
morning
afternoon
evening

The Relaxation Solution
Daily Journal

Today is _____

M T W T F S S

Theme of the Day

Exercises I Did
time — *duration* — *exercise* — *notes*

Tension I Observed
trigger — *emotion* — *body locations* — *resolution*

Relaxation Remembrance
trigger (sticker, red light...) — *working?*

Y N
Y N
Y N
Y N

Mood Check

morning

afternoon

evening

The Relaxation Solution
Daily Journal

Today is _____
M T W T F S S

Theme of the Day

Exercises I Did
time — *duration* — *exercise* — *notes*

Tension I Observed
trigger — *emotion* — *body locations* — *resolution*

Relaxation Remembrance
trigger (sticker, red light...) — *working?*

Y N
Y N
Y N
Y N

Mood Check
morning

afternoon

evening

The Relaxation Solution

Daily Journal

Today is _____

M T W T F S S

Theme of the Day

Exercises I Did

time	duration	exercise	notes

Tension I Observed

trigger	emotion	body locations	resolution

Relaxation Remembrance

trigger (sticker, red light...) — working?

- _____ Y N
- _____ Y N
- _____ Y N
- _____ Y N

Mood Check

morning
🙂 😐 🙁 😖 😒 😨

afternoon
🙂 😐 🙁 😖 😒 😨

evening
🙂 😐 🙁 😖 😒 😨

The Relaxation Solution
Daily Journal

Today is _____
M T W T F S S

Theme of the Day

Exercises I Did
time — *duration* — *exercise* — *notes*

Tension I Observed
trigger — *emotion* — *body locations* — *resolution*

Relaxation Remembrance
trigger (sticker, red light...) — *working?*

Y N
Y N
Y N
Y N

Mood Check

morning

afternoon

evening

The Relaxation Solution
Daily Journal

Today is _____
M T W T F S S

Theme of the Day

Exercises I Did
time — duration — exercise — notes

Tension I Observed
trigger — emotion — body locations — resolution

Relaxation Remembrance
trigger (sticker, red light...) — working?
Y N
Y N
Y N
Y N

Mood Check
morning
😊 😐 🙁 😣 ☹️ 😮

afternoon
😊 😐 🙁 😣 ☹️ 😮

evening
😊 😐 🙁 😣 ☹️ 😮

The Relaxation Solution
Daily Journal

Today is _____
M T W T F S S

Theme of the Day

Exercises I Did
time — *duration* — *exercise* — *notes*

Tension I Observed
trigger — *emotion* — *body locations* — *resolution*

Relaxation Remembrance
trigger (sticker, red light...) — *working?*

Y N
Y N
Y N
Y N

Mood Check
morning

afternoon

evening

The Relaxation Solution
Weekly Journal

Today is _____

M T W T F S S

Theme of the Week

Notes to Self

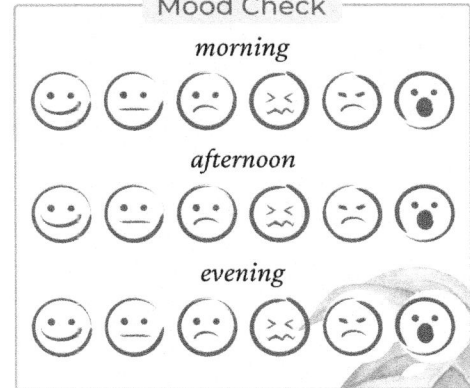

The Relaxation Solution
Daily Journal

Today is _____
M T W T F S S

Theme of the Day

Exercises I Did
time — *duration* — *exercise* — *notes*

Tension I Observed
trigger — *emotion* — *body locations* — *resolution*

Relaxation Remembrance
trigger (sticker, red light...) — *working?*

Y   N
Y   N
Y   N
Y   N

Mood Check
morning

afternoon

evening

The Relaxation Solution
Daily Journal

Today is _____

M T W T F S S

Theme of the Day

Exercises I Did
time — *duration* — *exercise* — *notes*

Tension I Observed
trigger — *emotion* — *body locations* — *resolution*

Relaxation Remembrance
trigger (sticker, red light...) — *working?*

Y N
Y N
Y N
Y N

Mood Check
morning

afternoon

evening

The Relaxation Solution
Daily Journal

Today is _____
M T W T F S S

Theme of the Day

Exercises I Did
time — *duration* — *exercise* — *notes*

Tension I Observed
trigger — *emotion* — *body locations* — *resolution*

Relaxation Remembrance
trigger (sticker, red light...) — *working?*

Y N
Y N
Y N
Y N

Mood Check
morning

afternoon

evening

The Relaxation Solution
Daily Journal

Today is _____

M T W T F S S

Theme of the Day

Exercises I Did
time — duration — exercise — notes

Tension I Observed
trigger — emotion — body locations — resolution

Relaxation Remembrance
trigger (sticker, red light...) — working?

Y N
Y N
Y N
Y N

Mood Check
morning

afternoon

evening

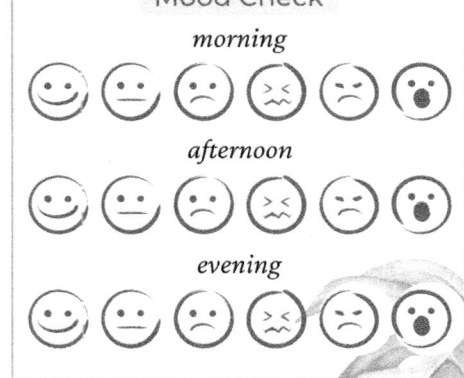

The Relaxation Solution
Daily Journal

Today is _____
M T W T F S S

Theme of the Day

Exercises I Did
time — *duration* — *exercise* — *notes*

Tension I Observed
trigger — *emotion* — *body locations* — *resolution*

Relaxation Remembrance
trigger (sticker, red light...) — *working?*

Y   N
Y   N
Y   N
Y   N

Mood Check
morning

afternoon

evening

The Relaxation Solution
Daily Journal

Today is _____
M T W T F S S

Theme of the Day

Exercises I Did
time — duration — exercise — notes

Tension I Observed
trigger — emotion — body locations — resolution

Relaxation Remembrance
trigger (sticker, red light...) — working?

Y N
Y N
Y N
Y N

Mood Check
morning

afternoon

evening

The Relaxation Solution
Daily Journal

Today is _____

M T W T F S S

Theme of the Day

Exercises I Did
time — *duration* — *exercise* — *notes*

Tension I Observed
trigger — *emotion* — *body locations* — *resolution*

Relaxation Remembrance
trigger (sticker, red light...) — *working?*

Y N
Y N
Y N
Y N

Mood Check

morning

afternoon

evening

The Relaxation Solution

Weekly Journal

Today is _____

M T W T F S S

Theme of the Week

Notes to Self

The Relaxation Solution
Monthly Self-Evaluation

Today is _____

M T W T F S S

Instructions

Thinking about your life during the past month, answer each question honestly. Don't try to add up specific events. Just respond with your impression or estimate. Write your answer in the *raw* column.

Answers

0 – never   1 – rarely   2 – sometimes   3 – often   4 – very often

Questions

answer: —— raw —— adj

1. How often have you been upset because of something that happened unexpectedly? ___ → ___
2. How often have you felt that you were unable to control the important things in your life? ___ → ___
3. How often have you felt nervous and stressed? ___ → ___
4. How often have you felt confident about your ability to handle your personal problems? ___ 4-↘ ___
5. How often have you felt that things were going your way? ___ 4-↘ ___
6. How often have you found that you could not cope with all the things that you had to do? ___ → ___
7. How often have you been able to control irritations in your life? ___ 4-↘ ___
8. How often have you felt that you were on top of things? ___ 4-↘ ___
9. How often have you been angered because of things that happened outside of your control? ___ → ___
10. How often have you felt difficulties were piling up so high you could not overcome them? ___ → ___

Total: ___

Scoring

Write an adjusted score in the *adj* column. To calculate *adj*:
For questions 4, 5, 7, and 8, subtract raw score from 4
(change 0 to 4, 1 to 3, 2 to 2, 3 to 1, and 4 to 0.)
For questions 1, 2, 3, 6, 9, and 10, copy the raw score into *adj*.

Evaluation

If your total adjusted score is...

0 to 13 - your stress level is **low**.
14 to 26 - your stress level is **moderate**.
27 to 40 - your stress level is **high**.

The Relaxation Solution
Daily Journal

Today is _____

M T W T F S S

Theme of the Day

Exercises I Did
time — duration — exercise — notes

Tension I Observed
trigger — emotion — body locations — resolution

Relaxation Remembrance
trigger (sticker, red light...) — working?

Y N
Y N
Y N
Y N

Mood Check
morning

afternoon

evening

The Relaxation Solution
Daily Journal

Today is _____

M T W T F S S

Theme of the Day

Exercises I Did
time — *duration* — *exercise* — *notes*

Tension I Observed
trigger — *emotion* — *body locations* — *resolution*

Relaxation Remembrance
trigger (sticker, red light...) — *working?*

Y N
Y N
Y N
Y N

Mood Check
morning

afternoon

evening

The Relaxation Solution
Daily Journal

Today is _____

M T W T F S S

Theme of the Day

Exercises I Did

time — duration — exercise — notes

Tension I Observed

trigger — emotion — body locations — resolution

Relaxation Remembrance

trigger (sticker, red light...) — *working?*

Y N
Y N
Y N
Y N

Mood Check

morning

afternoon

evening

The Relaxation Solution
Daily Journal

Today is _____

M T W T F S S

Theme of the Day

Exercises I Did
— time — duration — exercise — notes —

Tension I Observed
— trigger — emotion — body locations — resolution —

Relaxation Remembrance
— trigger (sticker, red light...) — working? —

Y N
Y N
Y N
Y N

Mood Check
morning

afternoon

evening

The Relaxation Solution
Daily Journal

Today is _____
M T W T F S S

Theme of the Day

Exercises I Did
time — duration — exercise — notes

Tension I Observed
trigger — emotion — body locations — resolution

Relaxation Remembrance
trigger (sticker, red light...) — working?

Y N
Y N
Y N
Y N

Mood Check
morning
😊 😐 🙁 😣 😒 😮

afternoon
😊 😐 🙁 😣 😒 😮

evening
😊 😐 🙁 😣 😒 😮

The Relaxation Solution
Daily Journal

Today is _____
M T W T F S S

Theme of the Day

Exercises I Did
time — *duration* — *exercise* — *notes*

Tension I Observed
trigger — *emotion* — *body locations* — *resolution*

Relaxation Remembrance
trigger (sticker, red light...) — *working?*

Y N
Y N
Y N
Y N

Mood Check
morning

afternoon

evening

The Relaxation Solution
Daily Journal

Today is _____
M T W T F S S

Theme of the Day

Exercises I Did
time — duration — exercise — notes

Tension I Observed
trigger — emotion — body locations — resolution

Relaxation Remembrance
trigger (sticker, red light...) — working?

Y N
Y N
Y N
Y N

Mood Check
morning

afternoon

evening

The Relaxation Solution

Weekly Journal

Today is _____

M T W T F S S

Theme of the Week

Notes to Self

The Relaxation Solution
Daily Journal

Today is _____

M T W T F S S

Theme of the Day

Exercises I Did
time — *duration* — *exercise* — *notes*

Tension I Observed
trigger — *emotion* — *body locations* — *resolution*

Relaxation Remembrance
trigger (sticker, red light...) — *working?*

Y   N
Y   N
Y   N
Y   N

Mood Check

morning

afternoon

evening

The Relaxation Solution
Daily Journal

Today is _____
M T W T F S S

Theme of the Day

Exercises I Did
time — duration — exercise — notes

Tension I Observed
trigger — emotion — body locations — resolution

Relaxation Remembrance
trigger (sticker, red light...) — working?

Y N
Y N
Y N
Y N

Mood Check
morning

afternoon

evening

The Relaxation Solution
Daily Journal

Today is _____

M T W T F S S

Theme of the Day

Exercises I Did

time — duration — exercise — notes

Tension I Observed

trigger — emotion — body locations — resolution

Relaxation Remembrance

trigger (sticker, red light...) — working?

Y N
Y N
Y N
Y N

Mood Check

morning

afternoon

evening

The Relaxation Solution
Daily Journal

Today is _____
M T W T F S S

Theme of the Day

Exercises I Did
time — *duration* — *exercise* — *notes*

Tension I Observed
trigger — *emotion* — *body locations* — *resolution*

Relaxation Remembrance
trigger (sticker, red light...) — *working?*

Y   N
Y   N
Y   N
Y   N

Mood Check

morning

afternoon

evening

The Relaxation Solution
Daily Journal

Today is _____
M T W T F S S

Theme of the Day

Exercises I Did
time — *duration* — *exercise* — *notes*

Tension I Observed
trigger — *emotion* — *body locations* — *resolution*

Relaxation Remembrance
trigger (sticker, red light...) — *working?*

Y   N
Y   N
Y   N
Y   N

Mood Check
morning
😊 😐 🙁 😖 😒 😮

afternoon
😊 😐 🙁 😖 😒 😮

evening
😊 😐 🙁 😖 😒 😮

The Relaxation Solution
Daily Journal

Today is _____
M T W T F S S

Theme of the Day

Exercises I Did
time — *duration* — *exercise* — *notes*

Tension I Observed
trigger — *emotion* — *body locations* — *resolution*

Relaxation Remembrance
trigger (sticker, red light...) — *working?*

Y N
Y N
Y N
Y N

Mood Check
morning

afternoon

evening

The Relaxation Solution
Daily Journal

Today is _____
M T W T F S S

Theme of the Day

Exercises I Did
time — *duration* — *exercise* — *notes*

Tension I Observed
trigger — *emotion* — *body locations* — *resolution*

Relaxation Remembrance
trigger (sticker, red light...) — *working?*

Y N
Y N
Y N
Y N

Mood Check
morning

afternoon

evening

The Relaxation Solution

Weekly Journal

Today is _____

M T W T F S S

Theme of the Week

Notes to Self

The Relaxation Solution
Daily Journal

Today is _____

M T W T F S S

Theme of the Day

Exercises I Did

time — *duration* — *exercise* — *notes*

Tension I Observed

trigger — *emotion* — *body locations* — *resolution*

Relaxation Remembrance

trigger (sticker, red light...) — *working?*

Y N
Y N
Y N
Y N

Mood Check

morning

afternoon

evening

The Relaxation Solution
Daily Journal

Today is _____
M T W T F S S

Theme of the Day

Exercises I Did
time *duration* *exercise* *notes*

Tension I Observed
trigger *emotion* *body locations* *resolution*

Relaxation Remembrance
trigger (sticker, red light...) *working?*

Y N
Y N
Y N
Y N

Mood Check
morning

afternoon

evening

The Relaxation Solution
Daily Journal

Today is _____
M T W T F S S

Theme of the Day

Exercises I Did
time — duration — exercise — notes

Tension I Observed
trigger — emotion — body locations — resolution

Relaxation Remembrance
trigger (sticker, red light...) — working?

Y N
Y N
Y N
Y N

Mood Check
morning
afternoon
evening

The Relaxation Solution
Daily Journal

Today is _____

M T W T F S S

Theme of the Day

Exercises I Did
time — *duration* — *exercise* — *notes*

Tension I Observed
trigger — *emotion* — *body locations* — *resolution*

Relaxation Remembrance
trigger (sticker, red light...) — *working?*

Y   N
Y   N
Y   N
Y   N

Mood Check
morning

afternoon

evening

The Relaxation Solution
Daily Journal

Today is _____
M T W T F S S

Theme of the Day

Exercises I Did
time — duration — exercise — notes

Tension I Observed
trigger — emotion — body locations — resolution

Relaxation Remembrance
trigger (sticker, red light...) — *working?*

Y N
Y N
Y N
Y N

Mood Check
morning

afternoon

evening

The Relaxation Solution
Daily Journal

Today is _____
M T W T F S S

Theme of the Day

Exercises I Did
time — *duration* — *exercise* — *notes*

Tension I Observed
trigger — *emotion* — *body locations* — *resolution*

Relaxation Remembrance
trigger (sticker, red light...) — *working?*

Y N
Y N
Y N
Y N

Mood Check
morning

afternoon

evening

The Relaxation Solution
Daily Journal

Today is _____
M T W T F S S

Theme of the Day

Exercises I Did
time — duration — exercise — notes

Tension I Observed
trigger — emotion — body locations — resolution

Relaxation Remembrance
trigger (sticker, red light...) — working?

Y N
Y N
Y N
Y N

Mood Check
morning

afternoon

evening

The Relaxation Solution
Weekly Journal

Today is _____

M T W T F S S

Theme of the Week

Notes to Self

The Relaxation Solution
Daily Journal

Today is _____
M T W T F S S

Theme of the Day

Exercises I Did
time — *duration* — *exercise* — *notes*

Tension I Observed
trigger — *emotion* — *body locations* — *resolution*

Relaxation Remembrance
trigger (sticker, red light...) — *working?*

Y N
Y N
Y N
Y N

Mood Check
morning

afternoon

evening

The Relaxation Solution
Daily Journal

Today is _____
M T W T F S S

Theme of the Day

Exercises I Did
time — *duration* — *exercise* — *notes*

Tension I Observed
trigger — *emotion* — *body locations* — *resolution*

Relaxation Remembrance
trigger (sticker, red light...) — *working?*

Y N
Y N
Y N
Y N

Mood Check
morning

afternoon

evening

The Relaxation Solution
Daily Journal

Today is _____

M T W T F S S

Theme of the Day

Exercises I Did
time — duration — exercise — notes

Tension I Observed
trigger — emotion — body locations — resolution

Relaxation Remembrance
trigger (sticker, red light...) — working?

Y N
Y N
Y N
Y N

Mood Check
morning

afternoon

evening

The Relaxation Solution
Daily Journal

Today is _____
M T W T F S S

Theme of the Day

Exercises I Did
time — *duration* — *exercise* — *notes*

Tension I Observed
trigger — *emotion* — *body locations* — *resolution*

Relaxation Remembrance
trigger (sticker, red light...) — *working?*

Y N
Y N
Y N
Y N

Mood Check
morning

afternoon

evening

The Relaxation Solution
Daily Journal

Today is _____
M T W T F S S

Theme of the Day

Exercises I Did
time — duration — exercise — notes

Tension I Observed
trigger — emotion — body locations — resolution

Relaxation Remembrance
trigger (sticker, red light...) — working?

Y N
Y N
Y N
Y N

Mood Check
morning

afternoon

evening

The Relaxation Solution
Daily Journal

Today is _____
M T W T F S S

Theme of the Day

Exercises I Did

time — *duration* — *exercise* — *notes*

Tension I Observed

trigger — *emotion* — *body locations* — *resolution*

Relaxation Remembrance

trigger (sticker, red light...) — *working?*

Y N
Y N
Y N
Y N

Mood Check

morning

afternoon

evening

The Relaxation Solution
Daily Journal

Today is _____

M T W T F S S

Theme of the Day

Exercises I Did
time — *duration* — *exercise* — *notes*

Tension I Observed
trigger — *emotion* — *body locations* — *resolution*

Relaxation Remembrance
trigger (sticker, red light...) — *working?*

Y N
Y N
Y N
Y N

Mood Check
morning

afternoon

evening

The Relaxation Solution
Weekly Journal

Today is _____

M T W T F S S

Theme of the Week

Notes to Self

The Relaxation Solution

Monthly Self-Evaluation

Today is _____

M T W T F S S

Instructions

Thinking about your life during the past month, answer each question honestly. Don't try to add up specific events. Just respond with your impression or estimate. Write your answer in the *raw* column.

Answers

0 – never   1 – rarely   2 – sometimes   3 – often   4 – very often

Questions

answer: raw   adj

1. How often have you been upset because of something that happened unexpectedly?   ___ → ___

2. How often have you felt that you were unable to control the important things in your life?   ___ → ___

3. How often have you felt nervous and stressed?   ___ → ___

4. How often have you felt confident about your ability to handle your personal problems?   ___ 4↺ ___

5. How often have you felt that things were going your way?   ___ 4↺ ___

6. How often have you found that you could not cope with all the things that you had to do?   ___ → ___

7. How often have you been able to control irritations in your life?   ___ 4↺ ___

8. How often have you felt that you were on top of things?   ___ 4↺ ___

9. How often have you been angered because of things that happened outside of your control?   ___ → ___

10. How often have you felt difficulties were piling up so high you could not overcome them?   ___ → ___

Total: ___

Scoring

Write an adjusted score in the *adj* column. To calculate *adj*:
For questions 4, 5, 7, and 8, subtract raw score from 4 (change 0 to 4, 1 to 3, 2 to 2, 3 to 1, and 4 to 0.)
For questions 1, 2, 3, 6, 9, and 10, copy the raw score into *adj*.

Evaluation

If your total adjusted score is...

0 to 13 - your stress level is **low**.
14 to 26 - your stress level is **moderate**.
27 to 40 - your stress level is **high**.

The Relaxation Solution
Daily Journal

Today is _____
M T W T F S S

Theme of the Day

Exercises I Did
time — *duration* — *exercise* — *notes*

Tension I Observed
trigger — *emotion* — *body locations* — *resolution*

Relaxation Remembrance
trigger (sticker, red light...) — *working?*

Y N
Y N
Y N
Y N

Mood Check
morning
afternoon
evening

The Relaxation Solution
Daily Journal

Today is _____

M T W T F S S

Theme of the Day

Exercises I Did
time *duration* *exercise* *notes*

Tension I Observed
trigger *emotion* *body locations* *resolution*

Relaxation Remembrance
trigger (sticker, red light...) *working?*

Y N
Y N
Y N
Y N

Mood Check
morning

afternoon

evening

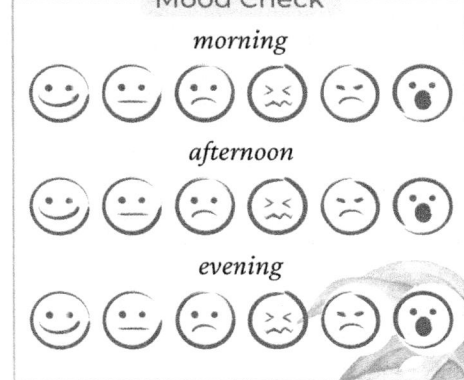

The Relaxation Solution
Daily Journal

Today is _____
M T W T F S S

Theme of the Day

Exercises I Did
— time — duration — exercise — notes —

Tension I Observed
— trigger — emotion — body locations — resolution —

Relaxation Remembrance
— trigger (sticker, red light...) — working? —

Y N
Y N
Y N
Y N

Mood Check
morning

afternoon

evening

The Relaxation Solution
Daily Journal

Today is _____
M T W T F S S

Theme of the Day

Exercises I Did
time — *duration* — *exercise* — *notes*

Tension I Observed
trigger — *emotion* — *body locations* — *resolution*

Relaxation Remembrance
trigger (sticker, red light...) — *working?*

Y N
Y N
Y N
Y N

Mood Check
morning

afternoon

evening

The Relaxation Solution
Daily Journal

Today is _____
M T W T F S S

Theme of the Day

Exercises I Did
time — *duration* — *exercise* — *notes*

Tension I Observed
trigger — *emotion* — *body locations* — *resolution*

Relaxation Remembrance
trigger (sticker, red light...) — *working?*

Y N
Y N
Y N
Y N

Mood Check
morning

afternoon

evening

The Relaxation Solution

Daily Journal

Today is _____

M T W T F S S

Theme of the Day

Exercises I Did

| time | duration | exercise | notes |

Tension I Observed

| trigger | emotion | body locations | resolution |

Relaxation Remembrance

trigger (sticker, red light...) — working?

- Y N
- Y N
- Y N
- Y N

Mood Check

morning

afternoon

evening

The Relaxation Solution
Daily Journal

Today is _____
M T W T F S S

Theme of the Day

Exercises I Did
time — *duration* — *exercise* — *notes*

Tension I Observed
trigger — *emotion* — *body locations* — *resolution*

Relaxation Remembrance
trigger (sticker, red light...) — *working?*

Y N
Y N
Y N
Y N

Mood Check
morning

afternoon

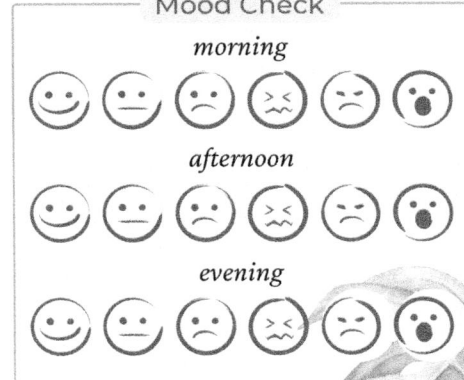

evening

The Relaxation Solution
Weekly Journal

Today is _____
M T W T F S S

Theme of the Week

Notes to Self

The Relaxation Solution
Daily Journal

Today is _____
M T W T F S S

Theme of the Day

Exercises I Did
time — *duration* — *exercise* — *notes*

Tension I Observed
trigger — *emotion* — *body locations* — *resolution*

Relaxation Remembrance
trigger (sticker, red light...) — *working?*

Y N
Y N
Y N
Y N

Mood Check
morning

afternoon

evening

The Relaxation Solution
Daily Journal

Today is _____
M T W T F S S

Theme of the Day

Exercises I Did
time — duration — exercise — notes

Tension I Observed
trigger — emotion — body locations — resolution

Relaxation Remembrance
trigger (sticker, red light...) — working?

Y   N
Y   N
Y   N
Y   N

Mood Check
morning
😊 😐 🙁 😣 😒 😮

afternoon
😊 😐 🙁 😣 😒 😮

evening
😊 😐 🙁 😣 😒 😮

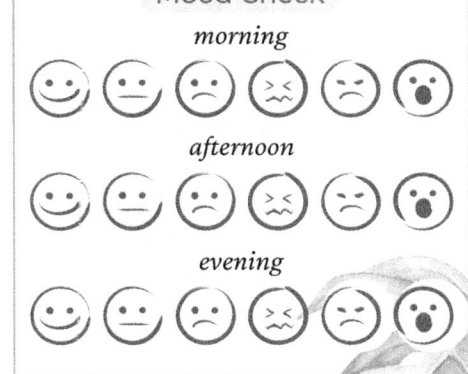

The Relaxation Solution
Daily Journal

Today is _____
M T W T F S S

Theme of the Day

Exercises I Did
time — *duration* — *exercise* — *notes*

Tension I Observed
trigger — *emotion* — *body locations* — *resolution*

Relaxation Remembrance
trigger (sticker, red light...) — working?
Y N
Y N
Y N
Y N

Mood Check
morning

afternoon

evening

The Relaxation Solution
Daily Journal

Today is _____

M T W T F S S

Theme of the Day

Exercises I Did
time — duration — exercise — notes

Tension I Observed
trigger — emotion — body locations — resolution

Relaxation Remembrance
trigger (sticker, red light...) — working?

Y N
Y N
Y N
Y N

Mood Check
morning

afternoon

evening

The Relaxation Solution
Daily Journal

Today is _____

M T W T F S S

Theme of the Day

Exercises I Did
time — *duration* — *exercise* — *notes*

Tension I Observed
trigger — *emotion* — *body locations* — *resolution*

Relaxation Remembrance
trigger (sticker, red light...) — *working?*

Y N
Y N
Y N
Y N

Mood Check
morning

afternoon

evening

The Relaxation Solution

Daily Journal

Today is _____
M T W T F S S

Theme of the Day

Exercises I Did
time — duration — exercise — notes

Tension I Observed
trigger — emotion — body locations — resolution

Relaxation Remembrance
trigger (sticker, red light...) — working?

- _____ Y N
- _____ Y N
- _____ Y N
- _____ Y N

Mood Check

morning

afternoon

evening

The Relaxation Solution
Daily Journal

Today is _____
M T W T F S S

Theme of the Day

Exercises I Did
time — *duration* — *exercise* — *notes*

Tension I Observed
trigger — *emotion* — *body locations* — *resolution*

Relaxation Remembrance
trigger (sticker, red light...) — *working?*

Y N
Y N
Y N
Y N

Mood Check
morning
afternoon
evening

The Relaxation Solution

Weekly Journal

Today is _____

M T W T F S S

---- Theme of the Week ----

---- Notes to Self ----

The Relaxation Solution
Daily Journal

Today is _____
M T W T F S S

Theme of the Day

Exercises I Did
time — *duration* — *exercise* — *notes*

Tension I Observed
trigger — *emotion* — *body locations* — *resolution*

Relaxation Remembrance
trigger (sticker, red light...) — *working?*

Y N
Y N
Y N
Y N

Mood Check
morning

afternoon

evening

The Relaxation Solution

Daily Journal

Today is _____

M T W T F S S

Theme of the Day

Exercises I Did

time   duration   exercise   notes

Tension I Observed

trigger   emotion   body locations   resolution

Relaxation Remembrance

trigger (sticker, red light…)   *working?*

Y   N
Y   N
Y   N
Y   N

Mood Check

morning

afternoon

evening

The Relaxation Solution
Daily Journal

Today is _____
M T W T F S S

Theme of the Day

Exercises I Did
time — *duration* — *exercise* — *notes*

Tension I Observed
trigger — *emotion* — *body locations* — *resolution*

Relaxation Remembrance
trigger (sticker, red light...) — *working?*

Y N
Y N
Y N
Y N

Mood Check
morning

afternoon

evening

The Relaxation Solution
Daily Journal

Today is _____

M T W T F S S

Theme of the Day

Exercises I Did
time — *duration* — *exercise* — *notes*

Tension I Observed
trigger — *emotion* — *body locations* — *resolution*

Relaxation Remembrance
trigger (sticker, red light...) — *working?*

Y N
Y N
Y N
Y N

Mood Check
morning

afternoon

evening

The Relaxation Solution
Daily Journal

Today is _____
M T W T F S S

Theme of the Day

Exercises I Did
time — *duration* — *exercise* — *notes*

Tension I Observed
trigger — *emotion* — *body locations* — *resolution*

Relaxation Remembrance
trigger (sticker, red light...) — *working?*

Y N
Y N
Y N
Y N

Mood Check
morning
afternoon
evening

The Relaxation Solution
Daily Journal

Today is _____

M T W T F S S

Theme of the Day

Exercises I Did
time — duration — exercise — notes

Tension I Observed
trigger — emotion — body locations — resolution

Relaxation Remembrance
trigger (sticker, red light...) — working?

Y N
Y N
Y N
Y N

Mood Check
morning

afternoon

evening

The Relaxation Solution
Daily Journal

Today is _____

M T W T F S S

Theme of the Day

Exercises I Did
time   *duration*   *exercise*   *notes*

Tension I Observed
trigger   *emotion*   *body locations*   *resolution*

Relaxation Remembrance
trigger (sticker, red light...)   *working?*

Y   N
Y   N
Y   N
Y   N

Mood Check
morning

afternoon

evening

The Relaxation Solution
Weekly Journal

Today is _____

M T W T F S S

Theme of the Week

Notes to Self

The Relaxation Solution
Daily Journal

Today is _____
M T W T F S S

Theme of the Day

Exercises I Did
time — *duration* — *exercise* — *notes*

Tension I Observed
trigger — *emotion* — *body locations* — *resolution*

Relaxation Remembrance
trigger (sticker, red light...) — *working?*

Y N
Y N
Y N
Y N

Mood Check
morning
afternoon
evening

The Relaxation Solution
Daily Journal

Today is _____
M T W T F S S

Theme of the Day

Exercises I Did
time — *duration* — *exercise* — *notes*

Tension I Observed
trigger — *emotion* — *body locations* — *resolution*

Relaxation Remembrance
trigger (sticker, red light...) — *working?*

Y N
Y N
Y N
Y N

Mood Check
morning

afternoon

evening

The Relaxation Solution
Daily Journal

Today is _____
M T W T F S S

Theme of the Day

Exercises I Did
time — *duration* — *exercise* — *notes*

Tension I Observed
trigger — *emotion* — *body locations* — *resolution*

Relaxation Remembrance
trigger (sticker, red light...) — *working?*

Y   N
Y   N
Y   N
Y   N

Mood Check
morning

afternoon

evening

The Relaxation Solution

Daily Journal

Today is _____

M T W T F S S

Theme of the Day

Exercises I Did

time	duration	exercise	notes

Tension I Observed

trigger	emotion	body locations	resolution

Relaxation Remembrance

trigger (sticker, red light...)	working?
	Y N
	Y N
	Y N
	Y N

Mood Check

morning

afternoon

evening

The Relaxation Solution
Daily Journal

Today is _____
M T W T F S S

Theme of the Day

Exercises I Did
time — *duration* — *exercise* — *notes*

Tension I Observed
trigger — *emotion* — *body locations* — *resolution*

Relaxation Remembrance
trigger (sticker, red light...) — *working?*

Y N
Y N
Y N
Y N

Mood Check
morning

afternoon

evening

The Relaxation Solution
Daily Journal

Today is _____

M T W T F S S

Theme of the Day

Exercises I Did

time — duration — exercise — notes

Tension I Observed

trigger — emotion — body locations — resolution

Relaxation Remembrance

trigger (sticker, red light...) — *working?*

Y N
Y N
Y N
Y N

Mood Check

morning

afternoon

evening

The Relaxation Solution
Daily Journal

Today is _____
M T W T F S S

Theme of the Day

Exercises I Did
time — *duration* — *exercise* — *notes*

Tension I Observed
trigger — *emotion* — *body locations* — *resolution*

Relaxation Remembrance
trigger (sticker, red light...) — *working?*

Y N
Y N
Y N
Y N

Mood Check
morning

afternoon

evening

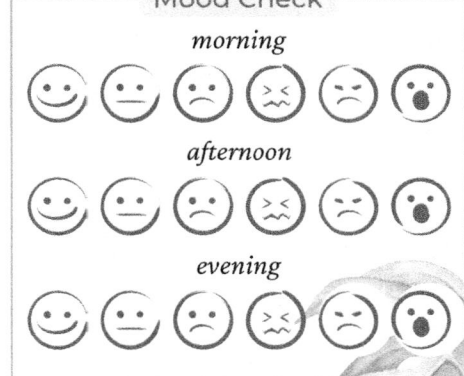

The Relaxation Solution
Weekly Journal

Today is _____

M T W T F S S

Theme of the Week

Notes to Self

The Relaxation Solution
Monthly Self-Evaluation

Today is _____

M T W T F S S

Instructions

Thinking about your life during the past month, answer each question honestly. Don't try to add up specific events. Just respond with your impression or estimate. Write your answer in the *raw* column.

Answers

0 – never   1 – rarely   2 – sometimes   3 – often   4 – very often

Questions

answer: — raw — adj

1. How often have you been upset because of something that happened unexpectedly? ___ → ___

2. How often have you felt that you were unable to control the important things in your life? ___ → ___

3. How often have you felt nervous and stressed? ___ → ___

4. How often have you felt confident about your ability to handle your personal problems? ___ 4-↘ ___

5. How often have you felt that things were going your way? ___ 4-↘ ___

6. How often have you found that you could not cope with all the things that you had to do? ___ → ___

7. How often have you been able to control irritations in your life? ___ 4-↘ ___

8. How often have you felt that you were on top of things? ___ 4-↘ ___

9. How often have you been angered because of things that happened outside of your control? ___ → ___

10. How often have you felt difficulties were piling up so high you could not overcome them? ___ → ___

Total: ___

Scoring

Write an adjusted score in the *adj* column. To calculate *adj*:
For questions 4, 5, 7, and 8, subtract raw score from 4
(change 0 to 4, 1 to 3, 2 to 2, 3 to 1, and 4 to 0.)
For questions 1, 2, 3, 6, 9, and 10, copy the raw score into *adj*.

Evaluation

If your total adjusted score is...

0 to 13 - your stress level is **low**.
14 to 26 - your stress level is **moderate**.
27 to 40 - your stress level is **high**.

The Relaxation Solution
Daily Journal

Today is _____

M T W T F S S

Theme of the Day

Exercises I Did
time — *duration* — *exercise* — *notes*

Tension I Observed
trigger — *emotion* — *body locations* — *resolution*

Relaxation Remembrance
trigger (sticker, red light...) — *working?*

Y N
Y N
Y N
Y N

Mood Check
morning
afternoon
evening

The Relaxation Solution
Daily Journal

Today is _____

M T W T F S S

Theme of the Day

Exercises I Did

time — *duration* — *exercise* — *notes*

Tension I Observed

trigger — *emotion* — *body locations* — *resolution*

Relaxation Remembrance

trigger (sticker, red light...) — *working?*

Y N
Y N
Y N
Y N

Mood Check

morning

afternoon

evening

The Relaxation Solution
Daily Journal

Today is _____
M T W T F S S

Theme of the Day

Exercises I Did
time — duration — exercise — notes

Tension I Observed
trigger — emotion — body locations — resolution

Relaxation Remembrance
trigger (sticker, red light...) — *working?*

Y N
Y N
Y N
Y N

Mood Check
morning
😊 😐 🙁 😣 😒 😮

afternoon
😊 😐 🙁 😣 😒 😮

evening
😊 😐 🙁 😣 😒 😮

The Relaxation Solution
Daily Journal

Today is _____
M T W T F S S

Theme of the Day

Exercises I Did
time — *duration* — *exercise* — *notes*

Tension I Observed
trigger — *emotion* — *body locations* — *resolution*

Relaxation Remembrance
trigger (sticker, red light...) — *working?*

Y N
Y N
Y N
Y N

Mood Check
morning

afternoon

evening

The Relaxation Solution
Daily Journal

Today is _____

M T W T F S S

Theme of the Day

Exercises I Did
time — duration — exercise — notes

Tension I Observed
trigger — emotion — body locations — resolution

Relaxation Remembrance
trigger (sticker, red light...) — *working?*

Y N
Y N
Y N
Y N

Mood Check
morning

afternoon

evening

The Relaxation Solution
Daily Journal

Today is _____
M T W T F S S

Theme of the Day

Exercises I Did
time — duration — exercise — notes

Tension I Observed
trigger — emotion — body locations — resolution

Relaxation Remembrance
trigger (sticker, red light...) — working?

Y N
Y N
Y N
Y N

Mood Check
morning

afternoon

evening

The Relaxation Solution
Daily Journal

Today is _____
M T W T F S S

Theme of the Day

Exercises I Did
time — duration — exercise — notes

Tension I Observed
trigger — emotion — body locations — resolution

Relaxation Remembrance
trigger (sticker, red light...) — working?

Y N
Y N
Y N
Y N

Mood Check
morning

afternoon

evening

The Relaxation Solution

Weekly Journal

Today is _____

M T W T F S S

Theme of the Week

Notes to Self

The Relaxation Solution
Daily Journal

Today is _____
M T W T F S S

Theme of the Day

Exercises I Did
time — *duration* — *exercise* — *notes*

Tension I Observed
trigger — *emotion* — *body locations* — *resolution*

Relaxation Remembrance
trigger (sticker, red light...) — *working?*

Y N
Y N
Y N
Y N

Mood Check
morning
afternoon
evening

The Relaxation Solution
Daily Journal

Today is _____
M T W T F S S

Theme of the Day

Exercises I Did
time — *duration* — *exercise* — *notes*

Tension I Observed
trigger — *emotion* — *body locations* — *resolution*

Relaxation Remembrance
trigger (sticker, red light...) — *working?*

Y N
Y N
Y N
Y N

Mood Check
morning

afternoon

evening

The Relaxation Solution
Daily Journal

Today is _____

M T W T F S S

Theme of the Day

Exercises I Did
time — duration — exercise — notes

Tension I Observed
trigger — emotion — body locations — resolution

Relaxation Remembrance
trigger (sticker, red light...) — working?

Y N
Y N
Y N
Y N

Mood Check
morning

afternoon

evening

The Relaxation Solution
Daily Journal

Today is _____
M T W T F S S

Theme of the Day

Exercises I Did
time — duration — exercise — notes

Tension I Observed
trigger — emotion — body locations — resolution

Relaxation Remembrance
trigger (sticker, red light...) — working?

Y N
Y N
Y N
Y N

Mood Check
morning

afternoon

evening

The Relaxation Solution
Daily Journal

Today is _____
M T W T F S S

Theme of the Day

Exercises I Did
time — *duration* — *exercise* — *notes*

Tension I Observed
trigger — *emotion* — *body locations* — *resolution*

Relaxation Remembrance
trigger (sticker, red light...) — *working?*

Y N
Y N
Y N
Y N

Mood Check
morning

afternoon

evening

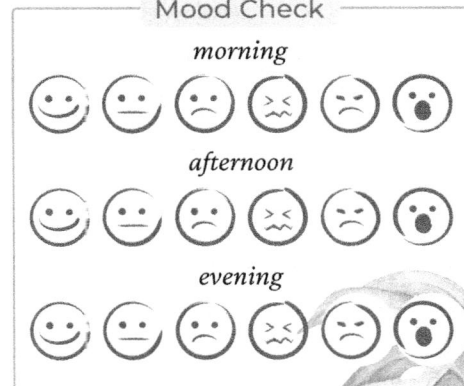

The Relaxation Solution
Daily Journal

Today is _____
M T W T F S S

Theme of the Day

Exercises I Did
time — duration — exercise — notes

Tension I Observed
trigger — emotion — body locations — resolution

Relaxation Remembrance
trigger (sticker, red light...) — working?

Y N
Y N
Y N
Y N

Mood Check
morning

afternoon

evening

The Relaxation Solution

Daily Journal

Today is _____

M T W T F S S

Theme of the Day

Exercises I Did

time — *duration* — *exercise* — *notes*

Tension I Observed

trigger — *emotion* — *body locations* — *resolution*

Relaxation Remembrance

trigger (sticker, red light...) — *working?*

Y   N
Y   N
Y   N
Y   N

Mood Check

morning

afternoon

evening

The Relaxation Solution

Weekly Journal

Today is _____

M T W T F S S

Theme of the Week

Notes to Self

The Relaxation Solution
Daily Journal

Today is _____
M T W T F S S

Theme of the Day

Exercises I Did
time — *duration* — *exercise* — *notes*

Tension I Observed
trigger — *emotion* — *body locations* — *resolution*

Relaxation Remembrance
trigger (sticker, red light...) — *working?*

Y N
Y N
Y N
Y N

Mood Check
morning

afternoon

evening

The Relaxation Solution
Daily Journal

Today is _____

M T W T F S S

Theme of the Day

Exercises I Did
time   *duration*   *exercise*   *notes*

Tension I Observed
trigger   *emotion*   *body locations*   *resolution*

Relaxation Remembrance
trigger (sticker, red light...)   *working?*

Y   N
Y   N
Y   N
Y   N

Mood Check
morning

afternoon

evening

The Relaxation Solution
Daily Journal

Today is _____

M T W T F S S

Theme of the Day

Exercises I Did
time — *duration* — *exercise* — *notes*

Tension I Observed
trigger — *emotion* — *body locations* — *resolution*

Relaxation Remembrance
trigger (sticker, red light...) — *working?*

Y N
Y N
Y N
Y N

Mood Check

morning

afternoon

evening

The Relaxation Solution
Daily Journal

Today is _____
M T W T F S S

Theme of the Day

Exercises I Did
time — duration — exercise — notes

Tension I Observed
trigger — emotion — body locations — resolution

Relaxation Remembrance
trigger (sticker, red light...) — working?

Y N
Y N
Y N
Y N

Mood Check
morning

afternoon

evening

The Relaxation Solution
Daily Journal

Today is _____
M T W T F S S

Theme of the Day

Exercises I Did
time — duration — exercise — notes

Tension I Observed
trigger — emotion — body locations — resolution

Relaxation Remembrance
trigger (sticker, red light…) — working?

- Y N
- Y N
- Y N
- Y N

Mood Check
morning

afternoon

evening

The Relaxation Solution
Daily Journal

Today is _____
M T W T F S S

Theme of the Day

Exercises I Did
time — duration — exercise — notes

Tension I Observed
trigger — emotion — body locations — resolution

Relaxation Remembrance
trigger (sticker, red light...) — *working?*

Y N
Y N
Y N
Y N

Mood Check
morning
afternoon
evening

The Relaxation Solution
Daily Journal

Today is _____

M T W T F S S

Theme of the Day

Exercises I Did
time — *duration* — *exercise* — *notes*

Tension I Observed
trigger — *emotion* — *body locations* — *resolution*

Relaxation Remembrance
trigger (sticker, red light...) — *working?*

Y N
Y N
Y N
Y N

Mood Check
morning

afternoon

evening

The Relaxation Solution

Weekly Journal

Today is _____

M T W T F S S

Theme of the Week

Notes to Self

The Relaxation Solution
Daily Journal

Today is _____
M T W T F S S

Theme of the Day

Exercises I Did
time — duration — exercise — notes

Tension I Observed
trigger — emotion — body locations — resolution

Relaxation Remembrance
trigger (sticker, red light...) — working?

Y N
Y N
Y N
Y N

Mood Check
morning

afternoon

evening

The Relaxation Solution
Daily Journal

Today is _____
M T W T F S S

Theme of the Day

Exercises I Did
time — *duration* — *exercise* — *notes*

Tension I Observed
trigger — *emotion* — *body locations* — *resolution*

Relaxation Remembrance
trigger (sticker, red light...) — *working?*

Y N
Y N
Y N
Y N

Mood Check
morning

afternoon

evening

The Relaxation Solution
Daily Journal

Today is _____
M T W T F S S

Theme of the Day

Exercises I Did
time — *duration* — *exercise* — *notes*

Tension I Observed
trigger — *emotion* — *body locations* — *resolution*

Relaxation Remembrance
trigger (sticker, red light...) — *working?*

Y N
Y N
Y N
Y N

Mood Check
morning

afternoon

evening

The Relaxation Solution
Daily Journal

Today is _____
M T W T F S S

Theme of the Day

Exercises I Did
time — *duration* — *exercise* — *notes*

Tension I Observed
trigger — *emotion* — *body locations* — *resolution*

Relaxation Remembrance
trigger (sticker, red light...) — *working?*

Y N
Y N
Y N
Y N

Mood Check
morning

afternoon

evening

The Relaxation Solution

Daily Journal

Today is _____

M T W T F S S

Theme of the Day

Exercises I Did

time	duration	exercise	notes

Tension I Observed

trigger	emotion	body locations	resolution

Relaxation Remembrance

trigger (sticker, red light...)   working?

Y   N

Y   N

Y   N

Y   N

Mood Check

morning

afternoon

evening

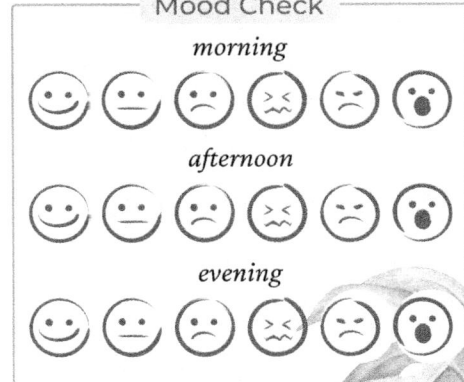

The Relaxation Solution
Daily Journal

Today is _____

M T W T F S S

Theme of the Day

Exercises I Did
time — *duration* — *exercise* — *notes*

Tension I Observed
trigger — *emotion* — *body locations* — *resolution*

Relaxation Remembrance
trigger (sticker, red light...) — *working?*

Y N
Y N
Y N
Y N

Mood Check

morning

afternoon

evening

The Relaxation Solution
Daily Journal

Today is _____

M T W T F S S

Theme of the Day

Exercises I Did

time — duration — exercise — notes

Tension I Observed

trigger — emotion — body locations — resolution

Relaxation Remembrance

trigger (sticker, red light...) — *working?*

Y N
Y N
Y N
Y N

Mood Check

morning

afternoon

evening

The Relaxation Solution

Weekly Journal

Today is _____

M T W T F S S

Theme of the Week

Notes to Self

The Relaxation Solution
Monthly Self-Evaluation

Today is _____
M T W T F S S

Instructions

Thinking about your life during the past month, answer each question honestly. Don't try to add up specific events. Just respond with your impression or estimate. Write your answer in the *raw* column.

Answers

0 – never   1 – rarely   2 – sometimes   3 – often   4 – very often

Questions

answer: raw   adj

1. How often have you been upset because of something that happened unexpectedly? →

2. How often have you felt that you were unable to control the important things in your life? →

3. How often have you felt nervous and stressed? →

4. How often have you felt confident about your ability to handle your personal problems? ↙4

5. How often have you felt that things were going your way? ↙4

6. How often have you found that you could not cope with all the things that you had to do? →

7. How often have you been able to control irritations in your life? ↙4

8. How often have you felt that you were on top of things? ↙4

9. How often have you been angered because of things that happened outside of your control? →

10. How often have you felt difficulties were piling up so high you could not overcome them? →

Total: ____

Scoring

Write an adjusted score in the *adj* column. To calculate *adj*:
For questions 4, 5, 7, and 8, subtract raw score from 4
(change 0 to 4, 1 to 3, 2 to 2, 3 to 1, and 4 to 0.)
For questions 1, 2, 3, 6, 9, and 10, copy the raw score into *adj*.

Evaluation

If your total adjusted score is...

0 to 13 - your stress level is **low**.
14 to 26 - your stress level is **moderate**.
27 to 40 - your stress level is **high**.

The Relaxation Solution
Daily Journal

Today is _____
M T W T F S S

Theme of the Day

Exercises I Did
time — *duration* — *exercise* — *notes*

Tension I Observed
trigger — *emotion* — *body locations* — *resolution*

Relaxation Remembrance
trigger (sticker, red light...) — *working?*

Y   N
Y   N
Y   N
Y   N

Mood Check
morning

afternoon

evening

The Relaxation Solution
Daily Journal

Today is _____
M T W T F S S

Theme of the Day

Exercises I Did
— time — duration — exercise — notes

Tension I Observed
— trigger — emotion — body locations — resolution

Relaxation Remembrance
— trigger (sticker, red light...) — working?

Y N
Y N
Y N
Y N

Mood Check
morning

afternoon

evening

The Relaxation Solution
Daily Journal

Today is _____

M T W T F S S

Theme of the Day

Exercises I Did
time — *duration* — *exercise* — *notes*

Tension I Observed
trigger — *emotion* — *body locations* — *resolution*

Relaxation Remembrance
trigger (sticker, red light...) — *working?*

Y N
Y N
Y N
Y N

Mood Check
morning

afternoon

evening

The Relaxation Solution
Daily Journal

Today is _____

M T W T F S S

Theme of the Day

Exercises I Did
time — duration — exercise — notes

Tension I Observed
trigger — emotion — body locations — resolution

Relaxation Remembrance
trigger (sticker, red light...) — working?

- Y N
- Y N
- Y N
- Y N

Mood Check
morning

afternoon

evening

The Relaxation Solution
Daily Journal

Today is _____
M T W T F S S

Theme of the Day

Exercises I Did
time — *duration* — *exercise* — *notes*

Tension I Observed
trigger — *emotion* — *body locations* — *resolution*

Relaxation Remembrance
trigger (sticker, red light...) — working?

Y N
Y N
Y N
Y N

Mood Check
morning

afternoon

evening

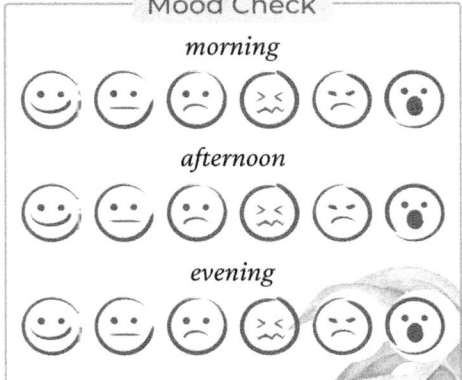

The Relaxation Solution
Daily Journal

Today is _____
M T W T F S S

Theme of the Day

Exercises I Did
time — *duration* — *exercise* — *notes*

Tension I Observed
trigger — *emotion* — *body locations* — *resolution*

Relaxation Remembrance
trigger (sticker, red light...) — *working?*

Y N
Y N
Y N
Y N

Mood Check
morning

afternoon

evening

The Relaxation Solution
Daily Journal

Today is _____
M T W T F S S

Theme of the Day

Exercises I Did
time — duration — exercise — notes

Tension I Observed
trigger — emotion — body locations — resolution

Relaxation Remembrance
trigger (sticker, red light...) — working?

Y N
Y N
Y N
Y N

Mood Check
morning
😊 😐 ☹️ 😖 😠 😮

afternoon
😊 😐 ☹️ 😖 😠 😮

evening
😊 😐 ☹️ 😖 😠 😮

The Relaxation Solution

Weekly Journal

Today is _____

M T W T F S S

Theme of the Week

Notes to Self

The Relaxation Solution
Daily Journal

Today is _____
M T W T F S S

Theme of the Day

Exercises I Did
time *duration* *exercise* *notes*

Tension I Observed
trigger *emotion* *body locations* *resolution*

Relaxation Remembrance
trigger (sticker, red light...) *working?*

Y N
Y N
Y N
Y N

Mood Check
morning

afternoon

evening

The Relaxation Solution
Daily Journal

Today is _____

M T W T F S S

Theme of the Day

Exercises I Did
time — *duration* — *exercise* — *notes*

Tension I Observed
trigger — *emotion* — *body locations* — *resolution*

Relaxation Remembrance
trigger (sticker, red light...) — *working?*

Y N
Y N
Y N
Y N

Mood Check

morning

afternoon

evening

The Relaxation Solution
Daily Journal

Today is _____

M **T** W T F S S

Theme of the Day

Exercises I Did

time — duration — exercise — notes

Tension I Observed

trigger — emotion — body locations — resolution

Relaxation Remembrance

trigger (sticker, red light...) — *working?*

Y N
Y N
Y N
Y N

Mood Check

morning

afternoon

evening

The Relaxation Solution
Daily Journal

Today is _____
M T W T F S S

Theme of the Day

Exercises I Did
time *duration* *exercise* *notes*

Tension I Observed
trigger *emotion* *body locations* *resolution*

Relaxation Remembrance
trigger (sticker, red light...) *working?*

Y N
Y N
Y N
Y N

Mood Check
morning

afternoon

evening

The Relaxation Solution
Daily Journal

Today is _____
M T W T F S S

Theme of the Day

Exercises I Did
time — *duration* — *exercise* — *notes*

Tension I Observed
trigger — *emotion* — *body locations* — *resolution*

Relaxation Remembrance
trigger (sticker, red light...) — *working?*

Y N
Y N
Y N
Y N

Mood Check
morning

afternoon

evening

The Relaxation Solution
Daily Journal

Today is _____

M T W T F S S

Theme of the Day

Exercises I Did
time — *duration* — *exercise* — *notes*

Tension I Observed
trigger — *emotion* — *body locations* — *resolution*

Relaxation Remembrance
trigger (sticker, red light...) — *working?*

Y   N
Y   N
Y   N
Y   N

Mood Check
morning

afternoon

evening

The Relaxation Solution
Daily Journal

Today is _____
M T W T F S S

Theme of the Day

Exercises I Did
time — *duration* — *exercise* — *notes*

Tension I Observed
trigger — *emotion* — *body locations* — *resolution*

Relaxation Remembrance
trigger (sticker, red light...) — *working?*

Y N
Y N
Y N
Y N

Mood Check

morning

afternoon

evening

The Relaxation Solution
Weekly Journal

Today is _____

M T W T F S S

Theme of the Week

Notes to Self

The Relaxation Solution
Daily Journal

Today is _____
M T W T F S S

Theme of the Day

Exercises I Did
time — *duration* — *exercise* — *notes*

Tension I Observed
trigger — *emotion* — *body locations* — *resolution*

Relaxation Remembrance
trigger (sticker, red light...) — *working?*

Y N
Y N
Y N
Y N

Mood Check
morning

afternoon

evening

The Relaxation Solution

Daily Journal

Today is _____
M T W T F S S

Theme of the Day

Exercises I Did
time — *duration* — *exercise* — *notes*

Tension I Observed
trigger — *emotion* — *body locations* — *resolution*

Relaxation Remembrance
trigger (sticker, red light...) — *working?*

Y   N
Y   N
Y   N
Y   N

Mood Check

morning

afternoon

evening

The Relaxation Solution
Daily Journal

Today is _____
M T W T F S S

Theme of the Day

Exercises I Did
time — *duration* — *exercise* — *notes*

Tension I Observed
trigger — *emotion* — *body locations* — *resolution*

Relaxation Remembrance
trigger (sticker, red light...) — *working?*

Y N
Y N
Y N
Y N

Mood Check
morning
afternoon
evening

The Relaxation Solution
Daily Journal

Today is _____

M T W T F S S

Theme of the Day

Exercises I Did
time — duration — exercise — notes

Tension I Observed
trigger — emotion — body locations — resolution

Relaxation Remembrance
trigger (sticker, red light...) — *working?*

Y N
Y N
Y N
Y N

Mood Check
morning

afternoon

evening

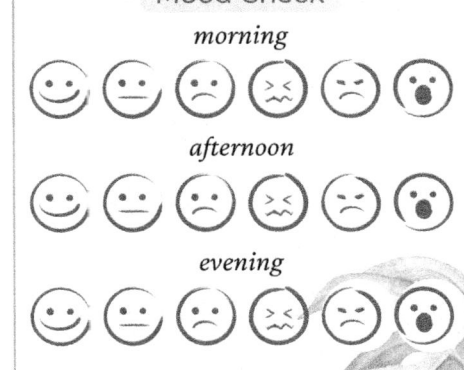

The Relaxation Solution
Daily Journal

Today is _____
M T W T F S S

Theme of the Day

Exercises I Did
time — duration — exercise — notes

Tension I Observed
trigger — emotion — body locations — resolution

Relaxation Remembrance
trigger (sticker, red light...) — working?

Y   N
Y   N
Y   N
Y   N

Mood Check
morning

afternoon

evening

The Relaxation Solution
Daily Journal

Today is _____

M T W T F S S

Theme of the Day

Exercises I Did
time — *duration* — *exercise* — *notes*

Tension I Observed
trigger — *emotion* — *body locations* — *resolution*

Relaxation Remembrance
trigger (sticker, red light...) — *working?*

Y   N
Y   N
Y   N
Y   N

Mood Check

morning

afternoon

evening

The Relaxation Solution
Daily Journal

Today is _____
M T W T F S S

Theme of the Day

Exercises I Did
time *duration* *exercise* *notes*

Tension I Observed
trigger *emotion* *body locations* *resolution*

Relaxation Remembrance
trigger (sticker, red light...) *working?*

Y N
Y N
Y N
Y N

Mood Check
morning

afternoon

evening

The Relaxation Solution
Weekly Journal

Today is _____
M T W T F S S

Theme of the Week

Notes to Self

The Relaxation Solution
Daily Journal

Today is _____
M T W T F S S

Theme of the Day

Exercises I Did
time — *duration* — *exercise* — *notes*

Tension I Observed
trigger — *emotion* — *body locations* — *resolution*

Relaxation Remembrance
trigger (sticker, red light...) — *working?*

Y N
Y N
Y N
Y N

Mood Check
morning

afternoon

evening

The Relaxation Solution
Daily Journal

Today is _____
M T W T F S S

Theme of the Day

Exercises I Did
time — *duration* — *exercise* — *notes*

Tension I Observed
trigger — *emotion* — *body locations* — *resolution*

Relaxation Remembrance
trigger (sticker, red light...) — *working?*

Y N
Y N
Y N
Y N

Mood Check
morning
😊 😐 ☹️ 😖 😒 😮

afternoon
😊 😐 ☹️ 😖 😒 😮

evening
😊 😐 ☹️ 😖 😒 😮

The Relaxation Solution
Daily Journal

Today is _____
M T W T F S S

Theme of the Day

Exercises I Did
time — *duration* — *exercise* — *notes*

Tension I Observed
trigger — *emotion* — *body locations* — *resolution*

Relaxation Remembrance
trigger (sticker, red light...) — *working?*

Y   N
Y   N
Y   N
Y   N

Mood Check
morning
😊 😐 🙁 😖 😠 😮

afternoon
😊 😐 🙁 😖 😠 😮

evening
😊 😐 🙁 😖 😠 😮

The Relaxation Solution
Daily Journal

Today is _____

M T W T F S S

Theme of the Day

Exercises I Did
time   *duration*   *exercise*   *notes*

Tension I Observed
trigger   *emotion*   *body locations*   *resolution*

Relaxation Remembrance
trigger (sticker, red light...)   *working?*

Y   N
Y   N
Y   N
Y   N

Mood Check
morning

afternoon

evening

The Relaxation Solution
Daily Journal

Today is _____

M T W T F S S

Theme of the Day

Exercises I Did
time — *duration* — *exercise* — *notes*

Tension I Observed
trigger — *emotion* — *body locations* — *resolution*

Relaxation Remembrance
trigger (sticker, red light...) — *working?*

Y N
Y N
Y N
Y N

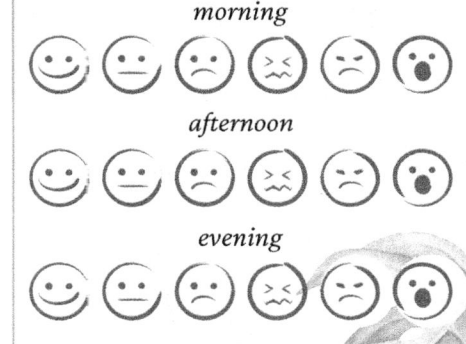

Mood Check

morning

afternoon

evening

The Relaxation Solution

Daily Journal

Today is _____
M T W T F S S

Theme of the Day

Exercises I Did

time	duration	exercise	notes

Tension I Observed

trigger	emotion	body locations	resolution

Relaxation Remembrance

trigger (sticker, red light...)	working?
	Y N
	Y N
	Y N
	Y N

Mood Check

morning
☺ 😐 ☹ 😖 😠 😮

afternoon
☺ 😐 ☹ 😖 😠 😮

evening
☺ 😐 ☹ 😖 😠 😮

The Relaxation Solution
Daily Journal

Today is _____
M T W T F S S

Theme of the Day

Exercises I Did
time — *duration* — *exercise* — *notes*

Tension I Observed
trigger — *emotion* — *body locations* — *resolution*

Relaxation Remembrance
trigger (sticker, red light...) — *working?*

Y N
Y N
Y N
Y N

Mood Check
morning

afternoon

evening

The Relaxation Solution

Weekly Journal

Today is _____

M T W T F S S

Theme of the Week

Notes to Self

The Relaxation Solution
Monthly Self-Evaluation

Today is _____

M T W T F S S

Instructions

Thinking about your life during the past month, answer each question honestly. Don't try to add up specific events. Just respond with your impression or estimate. Write your answer in the *raw* column.

Answers

0 – never   1 – rarely   2 – sometimes   3 – often   4 – very often

Questions

answer: —— raw —— adj

1. How often have you been upset because of something that happened unexpectedly? ___ → ___
2. How often have you felt that you were unable to control the important things in your life? ___ → ___
3. How often have you felt nervous and stressed? ___ → ___
4. How often have you felt confident about your ability to handle your personal problems? ___ 4-↘ ___
5. How often have you felt that things were going your way? ___ 4-↘ ___
6. How often have you found that you could not cope with all the things that you had to do? ___ → ___
7. How often have you been able to control irritations in your life? ___ 4-↘ ___
8. How often have you felt that you were on top of things? ___ 4-↘ ___
9. How often have you been angered because of things that happened outside of your control? ___ → ___
10. How often have you felt difficulties were piling up so high you could not overcome them? ___ → ___

Total: ___

Scoring

Write an adjusted score in the *adj* column. To calculate *adj*:
For questions 4, 5, 7, and 8, subtract raw score from 4
(change 0 to 4, 1 to 3, 2 to 2, 3 to 1, and 4 to 0.)
For questions 1, 2, 3, 6, 9, and 10, copy the raw score into *adj*.

Evaluation

If your total adjusted score is...

0 to 13 - your stress level is **low**.
14 to 26 - your stress level is **moderate**.
27 to 40 - your stress level is **high**.

The Relaxation Solution
Daily Journal

Today is _____

M T W T F S S

Theme of the Day

Exercises I Did
time — *duration* — *exercise* — *notes*

Tension I Observed
trigger — *emotion* — *body locations* — *resolution*

Relaxation Remembrance
trigger (sticker, red light...) — *working?*

Y N
Y N
Y N
Y N

Mood Check
morning

afternoon

evening

The Relaxation Solution
Daily Journal

Today is _____

M T W T F S S

Theme of the Day

Exercises I Did
time — *duration* — *exercise* — *notes*

Tension I Observed
trigger — *emotion* — *body locations* — *resolution*

Relaxation Remembrance
trigger (sticker, red light...) — *working?*

Y   N
Y   N
Y   N
Y   N

Mood Check

morning

afternoon

evening

The Relaxation Solution
Daily Journal

Today is ____
M T W T F S S

Theme of the Day

Exercises I Did
time — *duration* — *exercise* — *notes*

Tension I Observed
trigger — *emotion* — *body locations* — *resolution*

Relaxation Remembrance
trigger (sticker, red light...) — *working?*

Y N
Y N
Y N
Y N

Mood Check
morning

afternoon

evening

The Relaxation Solution
Daily Journal

Today is _____
M T W T F S S

Theme of the Day

Exercises I Did
time   *duration*   *exercise*   *notes*

Tension I Observed
trigger   *emotion*   *body locations*   *resolution*

Relaxation Remembrance
trigger (sticker, red light...)   *working?*

Y   N
Y   N
Y   N
Y   N

Mood Check
morning

afternoon

evening

The Relaxation Solution
Daily Journal

Today is _____
M T W T F S S

Theme of the Day

Exercises I Did
time — *duration* — *exercise* — *notes*

Tension I Observed
trigger — *emotion* — *body locations* — *resolution*

Relaxation Remembrance
trigger (sticker, red light...) — *working?*

Y N
Y N
Y N
Y N

Mood Check
morning

afternoon

evening

The Relaxation Solution
Daily Journal

Today is _____
M T W T F S S

Theme of the Day

Exercises I Did
time — *duration* — *exercise* — *notes*

Tension I Observed
trigger — *emotion* — *body locations* — *resolution*

Relaxation Remembrance
trigger (sticker, red light...) — *working?*

Y N
Y N
Y N
Y N

Mood Check
morning

afternoon

evening

The Relaxation Solution
Daily Journal

Today is _____

M T W T F S S

Theme of the Day

Exercises I Did
time — duration — exercise — notes

Tension I Observed
trigger — emotion — body locations — resolution

Relaxation Remembrance
trigger (sticker, red light...) — working?

Y N
Y N
Y N
Y N

Mood Check

morning

afternoon

evening

The Relaxation Solution

Weekly Journal

Today is _____

M T W T F S S

Theme of the Week

Notes to Self

The Relaxation Solution

Daily Journal

Today is _____

M T W T F S S

Theme of the Day

Exercises I Did

time	duration	exercise	notes

Tension I Observed

trigger	emotion	body locations	resolution

Relaxation Remembrance

trigger (sticker, red light...)   working?

- Y N
- Y N
- Y N
- Y N

Mood Check

morning

afternoon

evening

The Relaxation Solution
Daily Journal

Today is _____

M T W T F S S

Theme of the Day

Exercises I Did
time — *duration* — *exercise* — *notes*

Tension I Observed
trigger — *emotion* — *body locations* — *resolution*

Relaxation Remembrance
trigger (sticker, red light...) — *working?*

Y N
Y N
Y N
Y N

Mood Check
morning

afternoon

evening

The Relaxation Solution
Daily Journal

Today is _____
M T W T F S S

Theme of the Day

Exercises I Did
time   *duration*   *exercise*   *notes*

Tension I Observed
trigger   *emotion*   *body locations*   *resolution*

Relaxation Remembrance
trigger (sticker, red light...)   *working?*

Y   N
Y   N
Y   N
Y   N

Mood Check
morning

afternoon

evening

The Relaxation Solution
Daily Journal

Today is _____
M T W T F S S

Theme of the Day

Exercises I Did
time — *duration* — *exercise* — *notes*

Tension I Observed
trigger — *emotion* — *body locations* — *resolution*

Relaxation Remembrance
trigger (sticker, red light...) — *working?*

Y N
Y N
Y N
Y N

Mood Check
morning

afternoon

evening

The Relaxation Solution
Daily Journal

Today is _____
M T W T F S S

Theme of the Day

Exercises I Did
time — duration — exercise — notes

Tension I Observed
trigger — emotion — body locations — resolution

Relaxation Remembrance
trigger (sticker, red light...) — working?

Y N
Y N
Y N
Y N

Mood Check
morning

😊 😐 🙁 😣 😠 😮

afternoon

😊 😐 🙁 😣 😠 😮

evening

😊 😐 🙁 😣 😠 😮

The Relaxation Solution
Daily Journal

Today is _____

M T W T F S S

Theme of the Day

Exercises I Did
time — *duration* — *exercise* — *notes*

Tension I Observed
trigger — *emotion* — *body locations* — *resolution*

Relaxation Remembrance
trigger (sticker, red light...) — *working?*

Y N
Y N
Y N
Y N

Mood Check
morning

afternoon

evening

The Relaxation Solution
Daily Journal

Today is _____
M T W T F S S

Theme of the Day

Exercises I Did
time — *duration* — *exercise* — *notes*

Tension I Observed
trigger — *emotion* — *body locations* — *resolution*

Relaxation Remembrance
trigger (sticker, red light...) — *working?*

Y N
Y N
Y N
Y N

Mood Check
morning

afternoon

evening

The Relaxation Solution
Weekly Journal

Today is _____

M T W T F S S

Theme of the Week

Notes to Self

The Relaxation Solution
Daily Journal

Today is _____

M T W T F S S

Theme of the Day

Exercises I Did
time — *duration* — *exercise* — *notes*

Tension I Observed
trigger — *emotion* — *body locations* — *resolution*

Relaxation Remembrance
trigger (sticker, red light...) — *working?*

Y N
Y N
Y N
Y N

Mood Check
morning

afternoon

evening

The Relaxation Solution
Daily Journal

Today is _____
M T W T F S S

Theme of the Day

Exercises I Did
time — *duration* — *exercise* — *notes*

Tension I Observed
trigger — *emotion* — *body locations* — *resolution*

Relaxation Remembrance
trigger (sticker, red light...) — *working?*

Y N
Y N
Y N
Y N

Mood Check
morning

afternoon

evening

The Relaxation Solution
Daily Journal

Today is _____
M T W T F S S

Theme of the Day

Exercises I Did
time — duration — exercise — notes

Tension I Observed
trigger — emotion — body locations — resolution

Relaxation Remembrance
trigger (sticker, red light...) — working?

Y   N
Y   N
Y   N
Y   N

Mood Check
morning

afternoon

evening

The Relaxation Solution
Daily Journal

Today is _____
M T W T F S S

Theme of the Day

Exercises I Did
time — *duration* — *exercise* — *notes*

Tension I Observed
trigger — *emotion* — *body locations* — *resolution*

Relaxation Remembrance
trigger (sticker, red light...) — *working?*

Y N
Y N
Y N
Y N

Mood Check
morning

afternoon

evening

The Relaxation Solution
Daily Journal

Today is _____

M T W T F S S

Theme of the Day

Exercises I Did
time — duration — exercise — notes

Tension I Observed
trigger — emotion — body locations — resolution

Relaxation Remembrance
trigger (sticker, red light...) — working?

Y N
Y N
Y N
Y N

Mood Check
morning

afternoon

evening

The Relaxation Solution
Daily Journal

Today is _____
M T W T F S S

Theme of the Day

Exercises I Did
time — *duration* — *exercise* — *notes*

Tension I Observed
trigger — *emotion* — *body locations* — *resolution*

Relaxation Remembrance
trigger (sticker, red light...) — *working?*

Y N
Y N
Y N
Y N

Mood Check
morning

afternoon

evening

The Relaxation Solution
Daily Journal

Today is _____
M T W T F S S

Theme of the Day

Exercises I Did
time — duration — exercise — notes

Tension I Observed
trigger — emotion — body locations — resolution

Relaxation Remembrance
trigger (sticker, red light...) — *working?*

Y N
Y N
Y N
Y N

Mood Check
morning
afternoon
evening

The Relaxation Solution

Weekly Journal

Today is _____

M T W T F S S

Theme of the Week

Notes to Self

The Relaxation Solution
Daily Journal

Today is _____

M T W T F S S

Theme of the Day

Exercises I Did
time — *duration* — *exercise* — *notes*

Tension I Observed
trigger — *emotion* — *body locations* — *resolution*

Relaxation Remembrance
trigger (sticker, red light...) — *working?*

Y N
Y N
Y N
Y N

Mood Check

morning

afternoon

evening

The Relaxation Solution
Daily Journal

Today is _____
M T W T F S S

Theme of the Day

Exercises I Did
time — duration — exercise — notes

Tension I Observed
trigger — emotion — body locations — resolution

Relaxation Remembrance
trigger (sticker, red light...) — working?

Y N
Y N
Y N
Y N

Mood Check
morning

afternoon

evening

The Relaxation Solution
Daily Journal

Today is _____

M T W T F S S

Theme of the Day

Exercises I Did

time — duration — exercise — notes

Tension I Observed

trigger — emotion — body locations — resolution

Relaxation Remembrance

trigger (sticker, red light...) — working?

Y N
Y N
Y N
Y N

Mood Check

morning

afternoon

evening

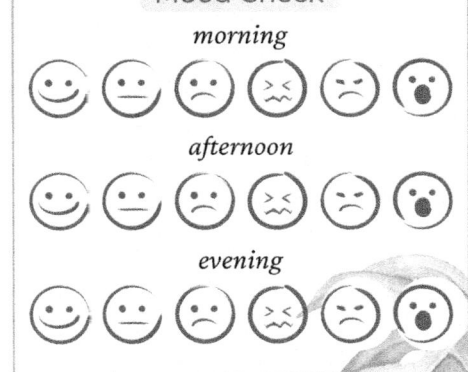

The Relaxation Solution
Daily Journal

Today is _____
M T W T F S S

Theme of the Day

Exercises I Did
time — *duration* — *exercise* — *notes*

Tension I Observed
trigger — *emotion* — *body locations* — *resolution*

Relaxation Remembrance
trigger (sticker, red light...) — *working?*

Y N
Y N
Y N
Y N

Mood Check
morning
😊 😐 🙁 😖 😣 😮

afternoon
😊 😐 🙁 😖 😣 😮

evening
😊 😐 🙁 😖 😣 😮

The Relaxation Solution
Daily Journal

Today is _____

M T W T F S S

Theme of the Day

Exercises I Did

time — *duration* — *exercise* — *notes*

Tension I Observed

trigger — *emotion* — *body locations* — *resolution*

Relaxation Remembrance

trigger (sticker, red light...) — *working?*

Y N
Y N
Y N
Y N

Mood Check

morning

afternoon

evening

The Relaxation Solution
Daily Journal

Today is _____
M T W T F S S

Theme of the Day

Exercises I Did
time — *duration* — *exercise* — *notes*

Tension I Observed
trigger — *emotion* — *body locations* — *resolution*

Relaxation Remembrance
trigger (sticker, red light...) — *working?*

Y N
Y N
Y N
Y N

Mood Check
morning

afternoon

evening

The Relaxation Solution
Daily Journal

Today is _____
M T W T F S S

Theme of the Day

Exercises I Did
time   *duration*   *exercise*   *notes*

Tension I Observed
trigger   *emotion*   *body locations*   *resolution*

Relaxation Remembrance
trigger (sticker, red light...)   *working?*

Y   N
Y   N
Y   N
Y   N

Mood Check
morning

afternoon

evening

The Relaxation Solution
Weekly Journal

Today is _____

M T W T F S S

Theme of the Week

Notes to Self

The Relaxation Solution
Monthly Self-Evaluation

Today is _____
M T W T F S S

Instructions

Thinking about your life during the past month, answer each question honestly. Don't try to add up specific events. Just respond with your impression or estimate. Write your answer in the *raw* column.

Answers

0 – never   1 – rarely   2 – sometimes   3 – often   4 – very often

Questions

answer: raw   adj

1. How often have you been upset because of something that happened unexpectedly? ___ → ___
2. How often have you felt that you were unable to control the important things in your life? ___ → ___
3. How often have you felt nervous and stressed? ___ → ___
4. How often have you felt confident about your ability to handle your personal problems? ___ 4↲ ___
5. How often have you felt that things were going your way? ___ 4↲ ___
6. How often have you found that you could not cope with all the things that you had to do? ___ → ___
7. How often have you been able to control irritations in your life? ___ 4↲ ___
8. How often have you felt that you were on top of things? ___ 4↲ ___
9. How often have you been angered because of things that happened outside of your control? ___ → ___
10. How often have you felt difficulties were piling up so high you could not overcome them? ___ → ___

Total: ___

Scoring

Write an adjusted score in the *adj* column. To calculate *adj*:
For questions 4, 5, 7, and 8, subtract raw score from 4 (change 0 to 4, 1 to 3, 2 to 2, 3 to 1, and 4 to 0.)
For questions 1, 2, 3, 6, 9, and 10, copy the raw score into *adj*.

Evaluation

If your total adjusted score is...

0 to 13 - your stress level is **low**.
14 to 26 - your stress level is **moderate**.
27 to 40 - your stress level is **high**.

The Relaxation Solution
Daily Journal

Today is _____

M T W T F S S

Theme of the Day

Exercises I Did

time — *duration* — *exercise* — *notes*

Tension I Observed

trigger — *emotion* — *body locations* — *resolution*

Relaxation Remembrance

trigger (sticker, red light...) — *working?*

Y N
Y N
Y N
Y N

Mood Check

morning

afternoon

evening

The Relaxation Solution
Daily Journal

Today is _____

M T W T F S S

Theme of the Day

Exercises I Did
time — duration — exercise — notes

Tension I Observed
trigger — emotion — body locations — resolution

Relaxation Remembrance
trigger (sticker, red light...) — working?

Y N
Y N
Y N
Y N

Mood Check
morning

afternoon

evening

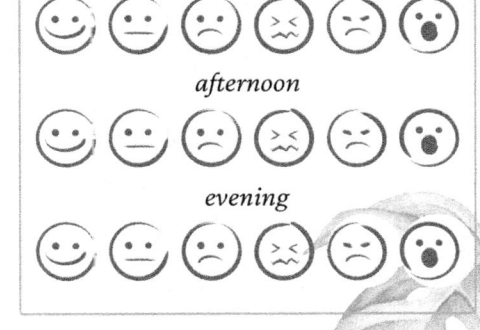

The Relaxation Solution
Daily Journal

Today is _____
M T W T F S S

Theme of the Day

Exercises I Did
time — *duration* — *exercise* — *notes*

Tension I Observed
trigger — *emotion* — *body locations* — *resolution*

Relaxation Remembrance
trigger (sticker, red light...) — *working?*

Y N
Y N
Y N
Y N

Mood Check
morning

afternoon

evening

The Relaxation Solution
Daily Journal

Today is _____
M T W T F S S

Theme of the Day

Exercises I Did
time — duration — exercise — notes

Tension I Observed
trigger — emotion — body locations — resolution

Relaxation Remembrance
trigger (sticker, red light...) — working?

Y N
Y N
Y N
Y N

Mood Check
morning
😊 😐 🙁 😣 😒 😮

afternoon
😊 😐 🙁 😣 😒 😮

evening
😊 😐 🙁 😣 😒 😮

The Relaxation Solution
Daily Journal

Today is _____
M T W T F S S

Theme of the Day

Exercises I Did
time — *duration* — *exercise* — *notes*

Tension I Observed
trigger — *emotion* — *body locations* — *resolution*

Relaxation Remembrance
trigger (sticker, red light...) — *working?*

Y N
Y N
Y N
Y N

Mood Check
morning

afternoon

evening

The Relaxation Solution

Daily Journal

Today is _____
M T W T F S S

Theme of the Day

Exercises I Did
time — duration — exercise — notes

Tension I Observed
trigger — emotion — body locations — resolution

Relaxation Remembrance
trigger (sticker, red light...) — *working?*

Y N
Y N
Y N
Y N

Mood Check
morning

afternoon

evening

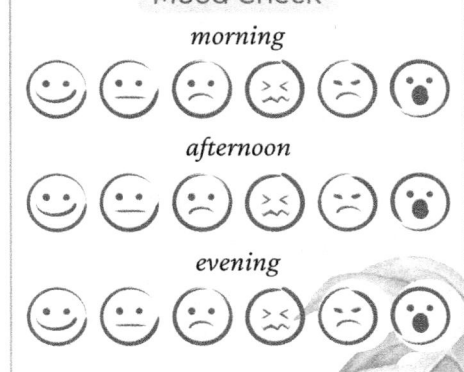

The Relaxation Solution
Daily Journal

Today is _____
M T W T F S S

Theme of the Day

Exercises I Did
time — *duration* — *exercise* — *notes*

Tension I Observed
trigger — *emotion* — *body locations* — *resolution*

Relaxation Remembrance
trigger (sticker, red light...) — *working?*

Y N
Y N
Y N
Y N

Mood Check
morning

afternoon

evening

The Relaxation Solution
Weekly Journal

Today is _____

M T W T F S S

Theme of the Week

Notes to Self

The Relaxation Solution
Daily Journal

Today is _____

M T W T F S S

Theme of the Day

Exercises I Did

time — *duration* — *exercise* — *notes*

Tension I Observed

trigger — *emotion* — *body locations* — *resolution*

Relaxation Remembrance

trigger (sticker, red light...) — *working?*

Y N
Y N
Y N
Y N

Mood Check

morning

afternoon

evening

The Relaxation Solution
Daily Journal

Today is _____

M T W T F S S

Theme of the Day

Exercises I Did
time *duration* *exercise* *notes*

Tension I Observed
trigger *emotion* *body locations* *resolution*

Relaxation Remembrance
trigger (sticker, red light...) *working?*

Y N
Y N
Y N
Y N

Mood Check
morning

afternoon

evening

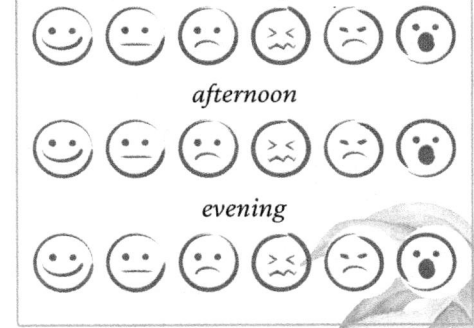

The Relaxation Solution
Daily Journal

Today is _____
M T W T F S S

Theme of the Day

Exercises I Did
time — *duration* — *exercise* — *notes*

Tension I Observed
trigger — *emotion* — *body locations* — *resolution*

Relaxation Remembrance
trigger (sticker, red light...) — *working?*

Y N
Y N
Y N
Y N

Mood Check
morning

afternoon

evening

The Relaxation Solution
Daily Journal

Today is _____
M T W T F S S

Theme of the Day

Exercises I Did
time —— duration —— exercise —————————— notes

Tension I Observed
trigger ————— emotion ————— body locations ————— resolution

Relaxation Remembrance
trigger (sticker, red light...) ———————— *working?*

Y N
Y N
Y N
Y N

Mood Check
morning

afternoon

evening

The Relaxation Solution
Daily Journal

Today is _____
M T W T F S S

Theme of the Day

Exercises I Did
time — *duration* — *exercise* — *notes*

Tension I Observed
trigger — *emotion* — *body locations* — *resolution*

Relaxation Remembrance
trigger (sticker, red light...) — *working?*

Y N
Y N
Y N
Y N

Mood Check
morning

afternoon

evening

The Relaxation Solution
Daily Journal

Today is _____

M T W T F S S

Theme of the Day

Exercises I Did
time — *duration* — *exercise* — *notes*

Tension I Observed
trigger — *emotion* — *body locations* — *resolution*

Relaxation Remembrance
trigger (sticker, red light...) — *working?*

Y N
Y N
Y N
Y N

Mood Check
morning

afternoon

evening

The Relaxation Solution
Daily Journal

Today is _____
M T W T F S S

Theme of the Day

Exercises I Did
time — *duration* — *exercise* — *notes*

Tension I Observed
trigger — *emotion* — *body locations* — *resolution*

Relaxation Remembrance
trigger (sticker, red light...) — *working?*

Y N
Y N
Y N
Y N

Mood Check
morning

afternoon

evening

The Relaxation Solution

Weekly Journal

Today is _____

M T W T F S S

Theme of the Week

Notes to Self

The Relaxation Solution
Daily Journal

Today is _____
M T W T F S S

Theme of the Day

Exercises I Did
time — duration — exercise — notes

Tension I Observed
trigger — emotion — body locations — resolution

Relaxation Remembrance
trigger (sticker, red light...) — working?

Y N
Y N
Y N
Y N

Mood Check
morning

afternoon

evening

The Relaxation Solution
Daily Journal

Today is _____
M T W T F S S

Theme of the Day

Exercises I Did
time *duration* *exercise* *notes*

Tension I Observed
trigger *emotion* *body locations* *resolution*

Relaxation Remembrance
trigger (sticker, red light...) *working?*

Y N
Y N
Y N
Y N

Mood Check
morning
afternoon
evening

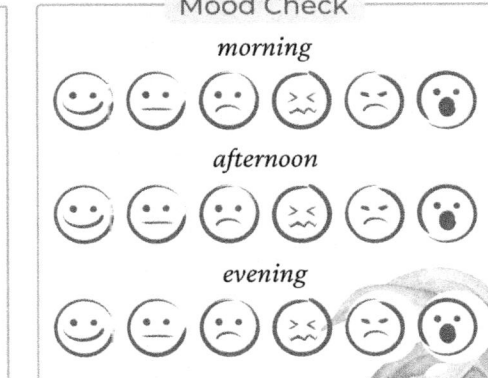

The Relaxation Solution
Daily Journal

Today is _____
M T W T F S S

Theme of the Day

Exercises I Did
time — *duration* — *exercise* — *notes*

Tension I Observed
trigger — *emotion* — *body locations* — *resolution*

Relaxation Remembrance
trigger (sticker, red light...) — *working?*

Y N
Y N
Y N
Y N

Mood Check
morning

afternoon

evening

The Relaxation Solution
Daily Journal

Today is _____
M T W T F S S

Theme of the Day

Exercises I Did
time — *duration* — *exercise* — *notes*

Tension I Observed
trigger — *emotion* — *body locations* — *resolution*

Relaxation Remembrance
trigger (sticker, red light...) — *working?*

Y N
Y N
Y N
Y N

Mood Check
morning
afternoon
evening

The Relaxation Solution
Daily Journal

Today is _____
M T W T F S S

Theme of the Day

Exercises I Did
time — duration — exercise — notes

Tension I Observed
trigger — emotion — body locations — resolution

Relaxation Remembrance
trigger (sticker, red light...) — working?

Y N
Y N
Y N
Y N

Mood Check
morning
afternoon
evening

The Relaxation Solution
Daily Journal

Today is _____
M T W T F S S

Theme of the Day

Exercises I Did
time — *duration* — *exercise* — *notes*

Tension I Observed
trigger — *emotion* — *body locations* — *resolution*

Relaxation Remembrance
trigger (sticker, red light...) — *working?*

Y N
Y N
Y N
Y N

Mood Check
morning

afternoon

evening

The Relaxation Solution
Daily Journal

Today is _____
M T W T F S S

Theme of the Day

Exercises I Did
time — *duration* — *exercise* — *notes*

Tension I Observed
trigger — *emotion* — *body locations* — *resolution*

Relaxation Remembrance
trigger (sticker, red light...) — *working?*

Y   N
Y   N
Y   N
Y   N

Mood Check
morning

afternoon

evening

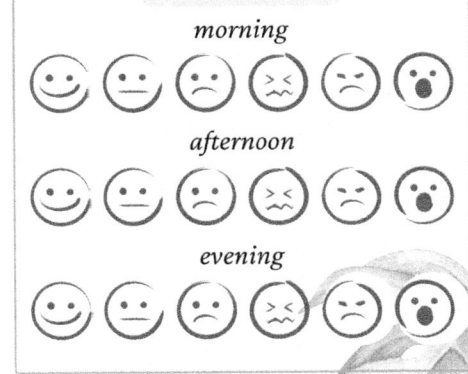

The Relaxation Solution
Weekly Journal

Today is _____

M T W T F S S

Theme of the Week

Notes to Self

The Relaxation Solution
Daily Journal

Today is _____
M T W T F S S

Theme of the Day

Exercises I Did
time — *duration* — *exercise* — *notes*

Tension I Observed
trigger — *emotion* — *body locations* — *resolution*

Relaxation Remembrance
trigger (sticker, red light...) — *working?*

Y N
Y N
Y N
Y N

Mood Check
morning

afternoon

evening

The Relaxation Solution
Daily Journal

Today is _____

M T W T F S S

Theme of the Day

Exercises I Did
time — duration — exercise — notes

Tension I Observed
trigger — emotion — body locations — resolution

Relaxation Remembrance
trigger (sticker, red light...) — working?

Y N
Y N
Y N
Y N

Mood Check
morning

afternoon

evening

The Relaxation Solution
Daily Journal

Today is _____
M T W T F S S

Theme of the Day

Exercises I Did
time — duration — exercise — notes

Tension I Observed
trigger — emotion — body locations — resolution

Relaxation Remembrance
trigger (sticker, red light...) — working?

Y N
Y N
Y N
Y N

Mood Check
morning

afternoon

evening

The Relaxation Solution
Daily Journal

Today is _____

M T W T F S S

Theme of the Day

Exercises I Did
time — *duration* — *exercise* — *notes*

Tension I Observed
trigger — *emotion* — *body locations* — *resolution*

Relaxation Remembrance
trigger (sticker, red light...) — *working?*

Y N
Y N
Y N
Y N

Mood Check
morning

afternoon

evening

The Relaxation Solution
Daily Journal

Today is _____

M T W T F S S

Theme of the Day

Exercises I Did

time — *duration* — *exercise* — *notes*

Tension I Observed

trigger — *emotion* — *body locations* — *resolution*

Relaxation Remembrance

trigger (sticker, red light...) — *working?*

Y N
Y N
Y N
Y N

Mood Check

morning

afternoon

evening

The Relaxation Solution
Daily Journal

Today is _____

M T W T F S S

Theme of the Day

Exercises I Did
time *duration* *exercise* *notes*

Tension I Observed
trigger *emotion* *body locations* *resolution*

Relaxation Remembrance
trigger (sticker, red light...) *working?*

Y N
Y N
Y N
Y N

Mood Check
morning

afternoon

evening

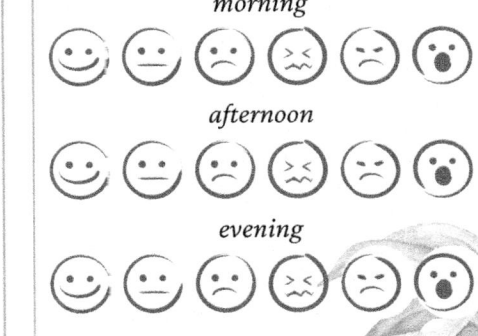

The Relaxation Solution
Daily Journal

Today is _____
M T W T F S S

Theme of the Day

Exercises I Did
time — *duration* — *exercise* — *notes*

Tension I Observed
trigger — *emotion* — *body locations* — *resolution*

Relaxation Remembrance
trigger (sticker, red light...) — *working?*

Y   N
Y   N
Y   N
Y   N

Mood Check
morning
afternoon
evening

The Relaxation Solution

Weekly Journal

Today is _____

M T W T F S S

Theme of the Week

Notes to Self

The Relaxation Solution
Monthly Self-Evaluation

Today is _____

M T W T F S S

Instructions

Thinking about your life during the past month, answer each question honestly. Don't try to add up specific events. Just respond with your impression or estimate. Write your answer in the *raw* column.

Answers

0 – never   1 – rarely   2 – sometimes   3 – often   4 – very often

Questions

answer: — raw — adj

1. How often have you been upset because of something that happened unexpectedly? ___ → ___

2. How often have you felt that you were unable to control the important things in your life? ___ → ___

3. How often have you felt nervous and stressed? ___ → ___

4. How often have you felt confident about your ability to handle your personal problems? ___ 4-↘ ___

5. How often have you felt that things were going your way? ___ 4-↘ ___

6. How often have you found that you could not cope with all the things that you had to do? ___ → ___

7. How often have you been able to control irritations in your life? ___ 4-↘ ___

8. How often have you felt that you were on top of things? ___ 4-↘ ___

9. How often have you been angered because of things that happened outside of your control? ___ → ___

10. How often have you felt difficulties were piling up so high you could not overcome them? ___ → ___

Total: ___

Scoring

Write an adjusted score in the *adj* column. To calculate *adj*:
For questions 4, 5, 7, and 8, subtract raw score from 4
(change 0 to 4, 1 to 3, 2 to 2, 3 to 1, and 4 to 0.)
For questions 1, 2, 3, 6, 9, and 10, copy the raw score into *adj*.

Evaluation

If your total adjusted score is…

0 to 13 - your stress level is **low**.
14 to 26 - your stress level is **moderate**.
27 to 40 - your stress level is **high**.

The Relaxation Solution
Daily Journal

Today is _____
M T W T F S S

Theme of the Day

Exercises I Did
time   *duration*   *exercise*   *notes*

Tension I Observed
trigger   *emotion*   *body locations*   *resolution*

Relaxation Remembrance
trigger (sticker, red light...)   *working?*

Y N
Y N
Y N
Y N

Mood Check
morning

afternoon

evening

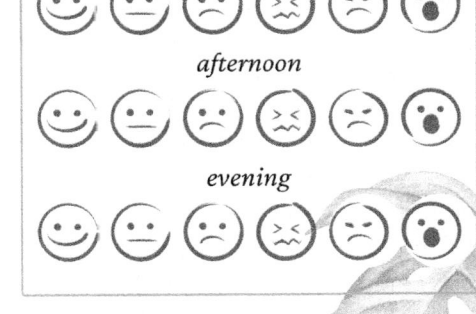

The Relaxation Solution
Daily Journal

Today is _____
M T W T F S S

Theme of the Day

Exercises I Did
time — *duration* — *exercise* — *notes*

Tension I Observed
trigger — *emotion* — *body locations* — *resolution*

Relaxation Remembrance
trigger (sticker, red light...) — *working?*

Y N
Y N
Y N
Y N

Mood Check
morning
afternoon
evening

The Relaxation Solution
Daily Journal

Today is _____
M T W T F S S

Theme of the Day

Exercises I Did
time — duration — exercise — notes

Tension I Observed
trigger — emotion — body locations — resolution

Relaxation Remembrance
trigger (sticker, red light...) — working?

Y N
Y N
Y N
Y N

Mood Check
morning
afternoon
evening

The Relaxation Solution
Daily Journal

Today is _____
M T W T F S S

Theme of the Day

Exercises I Did
time — *duration* — *exercise* — *notes*

Tension I Observed
trigger — *emotion* — *body locations* — *resolution*

Relaxation Remembrance
trigger (sticker, red light...) — *working?*

Y N
Y N
Y N
Y N

Mood Check
morning

afternoon

evening

The Relaxation Solution
Daily Journal

Today is _____

M T W T F S S

Theme of the Day

Exercises I Did
time — duration — exercise — notes

Tension I Observed
trigger — emotion — body locations — resolution

Relaxation Remembrance
trigger (sticker, red light...) — working?

	Y N
	Y N
	Y N
	Y N

Mood Check

morning
😊 😐 🙁 😣 😞 😮

afternoon
😊 😐 🙁 😣 😞 😮

evening
😊 😐 🙁 😣 😞 😮

The Relaxation Solution
Daily Journal

Today is ____
M T W T F S S

Theme of the Day

Exercises I Did
time — *duration* — *exercise* — *notes*

Tension I Observed
trigger — *emotion* — *body locations* — *resolution*

Relaxation Remembrance
trigger (sticker, red light...) — working?

Y N
Y N
Y N
Y N

Mood Check
morning

afternoon

evening

The Relaxation Solution
Daily Journal

Today is _____
M T W T F S S

Theme of the Day

Exercises I Did
time — *duration* — *exercise* — *notes*

Tension I Observed
trigger — *emotion* — *body locations* — *resolution*

Relaxation Remembrance
trigger (sticker, red light...) — *working?*

Y N
Y N
Y N
Y N

Mood Check
morning
afternoon
evening

The Relaxation Solution

Weekly Journal

Today is _____

M T W T F S S

Theme of the Week

Notes to Self

The Relaxation Solution
Daily Journal

Today is _____

M T W T F S S

Theme of the Day

Exercises I Did
time — *duration* — *exercise* — *notes*

Tension I Observed
trigger — *emotion* — *body locations* — *resolution*

Relaxation Remembrance
trigger (sticker, red light...) — *working?*

Y N
Y N
Y N
Y N

Mood Check
morning

afternoon

evening

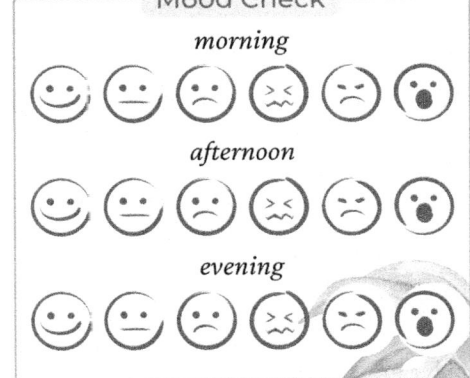

The Relaxation Solution
Daily Journal

Today is _____
M T W T F S S

Theme of the Day

Exercises I Did
time — *duration* — *exercise* — *notes*

Tension I Observed
trigger — *emotion* — *body locations* — *resolution*

Relaxation Remembrance
trigger (sticker, red light...) — *working?*

Y N
Y N
Y N
Y N

Mood Check
morning

afternoon

evening

The Relaxation Solution

Daily Journal

Today is _____

M T W T F S S

Theme of the Day

Exercises I Did

| time | duration | exercise | notes |

Tension I Observed

| trigger | emotion | body locations | resolution |

Relaxation Remembrance

trigger (sticker, red light...) — working?

Y N
Y N
Y N
Y N

Mood Check

morning
😊 😐 🙁 😖 😒 😮

afternoon
😊 😐 🙁 😖 😒 😮

evening
😊 😐 🙁 😖 😒 😮

The Relaxation Solution
Daily Journal

Today is _____
M T W T F S S

Theme of the Day

Exercises I Did
time — *duration* — *exercise* — *notes*

Tension I Observed
trigger — *emotion* — *body locations* — *resolution*

Relaxation Remembrance
trigger (sticker, red light...) — *working?*

Y N
Y N
Y N
Y N

Mood Check
morning
afternoon
evening

The Relaxation Solution
Daily Journal

Today is _____

M T W T F S S

Theme of the Day

Exercises I Did
time — *duration* — *exercise* — *notes*

Tension I Observed
trigger — *emotion* — *body locations* — *resolution*

Relaxation Remembrance
trigger (sticker, red light...) — *working?*

Y N
Y N
Y N
Y N

Mood Check
morning

afternoon

evening

The Relaxation Solution
Daily Journal

Today is _____
M T W T F S S

Theme of the Day

Exercises I Did
time — duration — exercise — notes

Tension I Observed
trigger — emotion — body locations — resolution

Relaxation Remembrance
trigger (sticker, red light...) — working?

Y   N
Y   N
Y   N
Y   N

Mood Check
morning

afternoon

evening

The Relaxation Solution

Daily Journal

Today is _____

M T W T F S S

Theme of the Day

Exercises I Did

time — *duration* — *exercise* — *notes*

Tension I Observed

trigger — *emotion* — *body locations* — *resolution*

Relaxation Remembrance

trigger (sticker, red light...) — *working?*

Y N
Y N
Y N
Y N

Mood Check

morning

afternoon

evening

The Relaxation Solution

Weekly Journal

Today is _____

M T W T F S S

Theme of the Week

Notes to Self

The Relaxation Solution
Daily Journal

Today is _____

M T W T F S S

Theme of the Day

Exercises I Did
time — duration — exercise — notes

Tension I Observed
trigger — emotion — body locations — resolution

Relaxation Remembrance
trigger (sticker, red light...) — *working?*

Y   N
Y   N
Y   N
Y   N

Mood Check
morning

afternoon

evening

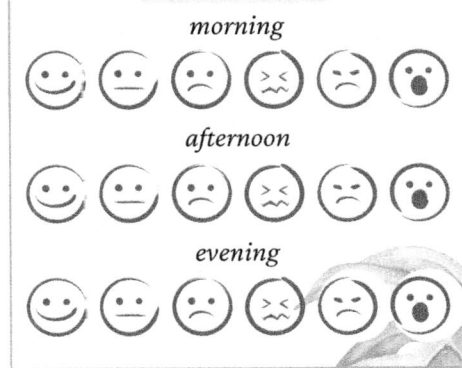

The Relaxation Solution
Daily Journal

Today is _____
M T W T F S S

Theme of the Day

Exercises I Did
time — *duration* — *exercise* — *notes*

Tension I Observed
trigger — *emotion* — *body locations* — *resolution*

Relaxation Remembrance
trigger (sticker, red light...) — *working?*

Y N
Y N
Y N
Y N

Mood Check
morning

afternoon

evening

The Relaxation Solution
Daily Journal

Today is _____

M T W T F S S

Theme of the Day

Exercises I Did
time — *duration* — *exercise* — *notes*

Tension I Observed
trigger — *emotion* — *body locations* — *resolution*

Relaxation Remembrance
trigger (sticker, red light...) — *working?*

Y N
Y N
Y N
Y N

Mood Check
morning

afternoon

evening

The Relaxation Solution
Daily Journal

Today is _____
M T W T F S S

Theme of the Day

Exercises I Did
time — duration — exercise — notes

Tension I Observed
trigger — emotion — body locations — resolution

Relaxation Remembrance
trigger (sticker, red light...) — working?

Y N
Y N
Y N
Y N

Mood Check
morning

afternoon

evening

The Relaxation Solution
Daily Journal

Today is _____
M T W T F S S

Theme of the Day

Exercises I Did
time — *duration* — *exercise* — *notes*

Tension I Observed
trigger — *emotion* — *body locations* — *resolution*

Relaxation Remembrance
trigger (sticker, red light...) — *working?*

Y N
Y N
Y N
Y N

Mood Check
morning

afternoon

evening

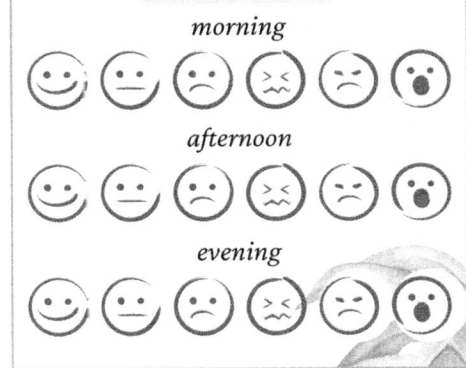

The Relaxation Solution
Daily Journal

Today is _____
M T W T F S S

Theme of the Day

Exercises I Did
time — *duration* — *exercise* — *notes*

Tension I Observed
trigger — *emotion* — *body locations* — *resolution*

Relaxation Remembrance
trigger (sticker, red light...) — *working?*

Y N
Y N
Y N
Y N

Mood Check
morning

afternoon

evening

The Relaxation Solution
Daily Journal

Today is _____
M T W T F S S

Theme of the Day

Exercises I Did
time — duration — exercise — notes

Tension I Observed
trigger — emotion — body locations — resolution

Relaxation Remembrance
trigger (sticker, red light...) — working?

Y N
Y N
Y N
Y N

Mood Check
morning

afternoon

evening

The Relaxation Solution
Weekly Journal

Today is _____

M T W T F S S

Theme of the Week

Notes to Self

The Relaxation Solution
Daily Journal

Today is _____

M T W T F S S

Theme of the Day

Exercises I Did

time — duration — exercise — notes

Tension I Observed

trigger — emotion — body locations — resolution

Relaxation Remembrance

trigger (sticker, red light...) — *working?*

Y N
Y N
Y N
Y N

Mood Check

morning

afternoon

evening

The Relaxation Solution
Daily Journal

Today is _____

M T W T F S S

Theme of the Day

Exercises I Did

time	duration	exercise	notes

Tension I Observed

trigger	emotion	body locations	resolution

Relaxation Remembrance

trigger (sticker, red light...)   working?

- Y N
- Y N
- Y N
- Y N

Mood Check

morning
😊 😐 🙁 😖 😒 😮

afternoon
😊 😐 🙁 😖 😒 😮

evening
😊 😐 🙁 😖 😒 😮

The Relaxation Solution
Daily Journal

Today is _____
M T W T F S S

Theme of the Day

Exercises I Did
time — duration — exercise — notes

Tension I Observed
trigger — emotion — body locations — resolution

Relaxation Remembrance
trigger (sticker, red light...) — working?

Y N
Y N
Y N
Y N

Mood Check
morning

afternoon

evening

The Relaxation Solution
Daily Journal

Today is _____
M T W T F S S

Theme of the Day

Exercises I Did
time — *duration* — *exercise* — *notes*

Tension I Observed
trigger — *emotion* — *body locations* — *resolution*

Relaxation Remembrance
trigger (sticker, red light...) — *working?*

Y N
Y N
Y N
Y N

Mood Check
morning

afternoon

evening

The Relaxation Solution
Daily Journal

Today is _____

M T W T F S S

Theme of the Day

Exercises I Did
time — duration — exercise — notes

Tension I Observed
trigger — emotion — body locations — resolution

Relaxation Remembrance
trigger (sticker, red light...) — working?

Y N
Y N
Y N
Y N

Mood Check
morning

afternoon

evening

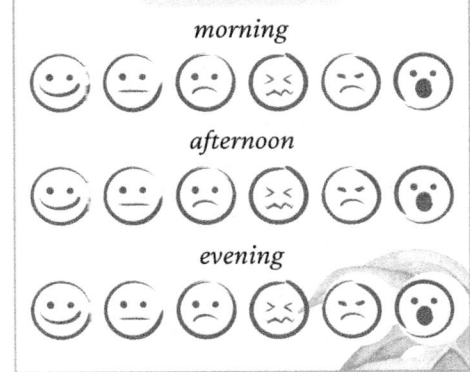

The Relaxation Solution
Daily Journal

Today is _____
M T W T F S S

Theme of the Day

Exercises I Did
time — *duration* — *exercise* — *notes*

Tension I Observed
trigger — *emotion* — *body locations* — *resolution*

Relaxation Remembrance
trigger (sticker, red light...) — working?

Y N
Y N
Y N
Y N

Mood Check
morning

afternoon

evening

The Relaxation Solution
Daily Journal

Today is _____
M T W T F S S

Theme of the Day

Exercises I Did
time — duration — exercise — notes

Tension I Observed
trigger — emotion — body locations — resolution

Relaxation Remembrance
trigger (sticker, red light...) — working?

Y N
Y N
Y N
Y N

Mood Check
morning

afternoon

evening

The Relaxation Solution

Weekly Journal

Today is _____

M T W T F S S

Theme of the Week

Notes to Self

The Relaxation Solution
Monthly Self-Evaluation

Today is _____

M T W T F S S

Instructions

Thinking about your life during the past month, answer each question honestly. Don't try to add up specific events. Just respond with your impression or estimate. Write your answer in the *raw* column.

Answers

0 – never   1 – rarely   2 – sometimes   3 – often   4 – very often

Questions

answer: ——— raw ——— adj

1. How often have you been upset because of something that happened unexpectedly? ___ → ___

2. How often have you felt that you were unable to control the important things in your life? ___ → ___

3. How often have you felt nervous and stressed? ___ → ___

4. How often have you felt confident about your ability to handle your personal problems? ___ 4-↘ ___

5. How often have you felt that things were going your way? ___ 4-↘ ___

6. How often have you found that you could not cope with all the things that you had to do? ___ → ___

7. How often have you been able to control irritations in your life? ___ 4-↘ ___

8. How often have you felt that you were on top of things? ___ 4-↘ ___

9. How often have you been angered because of things that happened outside of your control? ___ → ___

10. How often have you felt difficulties were piling up so high you could not overcome them? ___ → ___

Total: ___

Scoring

Write an adjusted score in the *adj* column. To calculate *adj*:
For questions 4, 5, 7, and 8, subtract raw score from 4 (change 0 to 4, 1 to 3, 2 to 2, 3 to 1, and 4 to 0.)
For questions 1, 2, 3, 6, 9, and 10, copy the raw score into *adj*.

Evaluation

If your total adjusted score is...

0 to 13 - your stress level is **low**.
14 to 26 - your stress level is **moderate**.
27 to 40 - your stress level is **high**.

The Relaxation Solution
Daily Journal

Today is _____

M T W T F S S

Theme of the Day

Exercises I Did

time — *duration* — *exercise* — *notes*

Tension I Observed

trigger — *emotion* — *body locations* — *resolution*

Relaxation Remembrance

trigger (sticker, red light...) — *working?*

Y N
Y N
Y N
Y N

Mood Check

morning

afternoon

evening

The Relaxation Solution
Daily Journal

Today is _____

M T W T F S S

Theme of the Day

Exercises I Did
time — *duration* — *exercise* — *notes*

Tension I Observed
trigger — *emotion* — *body locations* — *resolution*

Relaxation Remembrance
trigger (sticker, red light...) — *working?*

Y N
Y N
Y N
Y N

Mood Check
morning

afternoon

evening

The Relaxation Solution
Daily Journal

Today is _____
M T W T F S S

Theme of the Day

Exercises I Did
time — duration — exercise — notes

Tension I Observed
trigger — emotion — body locations — resolution

Relaxation Remembrance
trigger (sticker, red light...) — working?

Y N
Y N
Y N
Y N

Mood Check
morning

afternoon

evening

The Relaxation Solution
Daily Journal

Today is _____
M T W T F S S

Theme of the Day

Exercises I Did
time — duration — exercise — notes

Tension I Observed
trigger — emotion — body locations — resolution

Relaxation Remembrance
trigger (sticker, red light...) — *working?*

Y N
Y N
Y N
Y N

Mood Check
morning

afternoon

evening

The Relaxation Solution
Daily Journal

Today is _____
M T W T F S S

Theme of the Day

Exercises I Did
time — *duration* — *exercise* — *notes*

Tension I Observed
trigger — *emotion* — *body locations* — *resolution*

Relaxation Remembrance
trigger (sticker, red light…) — *working?*

Y N
Y N
Y N
Y N

Mood Check
morning

afternoon

evening

The Relaxation Solution
Daily Journal

Today is _____

M T W T F S S

Theme of the Day

Exercises I Did
time — *duration* — *exercise* — *notes*

Tension I Observed
trigger — *emotion* — *body locations* — *resolution*

Relaxation Remembrance
trigger (sticker, red light...) — *working?*

Y N
Y N
Y N
Y N

Mood Check
morning

afternoon

evening

The Relaxation Solution
Daily Journal

Today is _____
M T W T F S S

Theme of the Day

Exercises I Did
time — *duration* — *exercise* — *notes*

Tension I Observed
trigger — *emotion* — *body locations* — *resolution*

Relaxation Remembrance
trigger (sticker, red light...) — *working?*

Y N
Y N
Y N
Y N

Mood Check
morning

afternoon

evening

The Relaxation Solution
Weekly Journal

Today is _____
M T W T F S S

Theme of the Week

Notes to Self

The Relaxation Solution
Daily Journal

Today is _____
M T W T F S S

Theme of the Day

Exercises I Did
time — *duration* — *exercise* — *notes*

Tension I Observed
trigger — *emotion* — *body locations* — *resolution*

Relaxation Remembrance
trigger (sticker, red light...) — *working?*

Y N
Y N
Y N
Y N

Mood Check
morning

afternoon

evening

The Relaxation Solution
Daily Journal

Today is _____
M T W T F S S

Theme of the Day

Exercises I Did
time — *duration* — *exercise* — *notes*

Tension I Observed
trigger — *emotion* — *body locations* — *resolution*

Relaxation Remembrance
trigger (sticker, red light...) — *working?*

Y N
Y N
Y N
Y N

Mood Check
morning
☺ 😐 🙁 😖 😒 😮

afternoon
☺ 😐 🙁 😖 😒 😮

evening
☺ 😐 🙁 😖 😒 😮

The Relaxation Solution
Daily Journal

Today is _____
M T W T F S S

Theme of the Day

Exercises I Did
time — duration — exercise — notes

Tension I Observed
trigger — emotion — body locations — resolution

Relaxation Remembrance
trigger (sticker, red light...) — working?

Y N
Y N
Y N
Y N

Mood Check

morning

afternoon

evening

The Relaxation Solution
Daily Journal

Today is _____

M T W T F S S

Theme of the Day

Exercises I Did
time — *duration* — *exercise* — *notes*

Tension I Observed
trigger — *emotion* — *body locations* — *resolution*

Relaxation Remembrance
trigger (sticker, red light...) — *working?*

Y N
Y N
Y N
Y N

Mood Check
morning

afternoon

evening

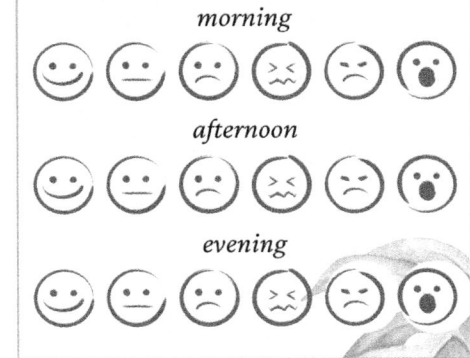

The Relaxation Solution
Daily Journal

Today is _____
M T W T F S S

Theme of the Day

Exercises I Did
time — *duration* — *exercise* — *notes*

Tension I Observed
trigger — *emotion* — *body locations* — *resolution*

Relaxation Remembrance
trigger (sticker, red light...) — *working?*

Y N
Y N
Y N
Y N

Mood Check
morning
😊 😐 🙁 😣 😒 😮

afternoon
😊 😐 🙁 😣 😒 😮

evening
😊 😐 🙁 😣 😒 😮

The Relaxation Solution
Daily Journal

Today is _____

M T W T F S S

Theme of the Day

Exercises I Did
time — *duration* — *exercise* — *notes*

Tension I Observed
trigger — *emotion* — *body locations* — *resolution*

Relaxation Remembrance
trigger (sticker, red light...) — *working?*

Y N
Y N
Y N
Y N

Mood Check
morning

afternoon

evening

The Relaxation Solution
Daily Journal

Today is _____
M T W T F S S

Theme of the Day

Exercises I Did
time *duration* *exercise* *notes*

Tension I Observed
trigger *emotion* *body locations* *resolution*

Relaxation Remembrance
trigger (sticker, red light...) *working?*

Y N
Y N
Y N
Y N

Mood Check
morning

afternoon

evening

The Relaxation Solution

Weekly Journal

Today is _____

M T W T F S S

Theme of the Week

Notes to Self

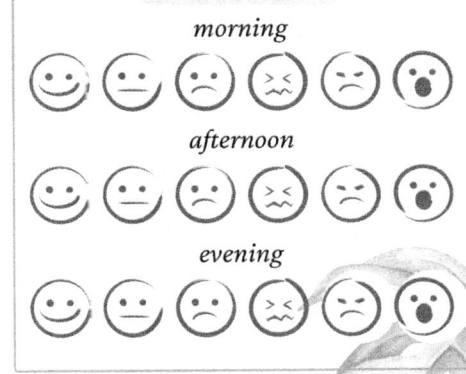

The Relaxation Solution
Daily Journal

Today is _____
M T W T F S S

Theme of the Day

Exercises I Did
time — *duration* — *exercise* — *notes*

Tension I Observed
trigger — *emotion* — *body locations* — *resolution*

Relaxation Remembrance
trigger (sticker, red light…) — *working?*

Y N
Y N
Y N
Y N

Mood Check
morning

afternoon

evening

The Relaxation Solution
Daily Journal

Today is _____
M T W T F S S

Theme of the Day

Exercises I Did
time — duration — exercise — notes

Tension I Observed
trigger — emotion — body locations — resolution

Relaxation Remembrance
trigger (sticker, red light...) — working?

Y N
Y N
Y N
Y N

Mood Check
morning

afternoon

evening

The Relaxation Solution
Daily Journal

Today is _____
M T W T F S S

Theme of the Day

Exercises I Did
time *duration* *exercise* *notes*

Tension I Observed
trigger *emotion* *body locations* *resolution*

Relaxation Remembrance
trigger (sticker, red light...) *working?*

Y N
Y N
Y N
Y N

Mood Check
morning

afternoon

evening

The Relaxation Solution
Daily Journal

Today is _____

M T W T F S S

Theme of the Day

Exercises I Did
time — *duration* — *exercise* — *notes*

Tension I Observed
trigger — *emotion* — *body locations* — *resolution*

Relaxation Remembrance
trigger (sticker, red light...) — *working?*

Y N
Y N
Y N
Y N

Mood Check
morning

afternoon

evening

The Relaxation Solution
Daily Journal

Today is _____
M T W T F S S

Theme of the Day

Exercises I Did
time — *duration* — *exercise* — *notes*

Tension I Observed
trigger — *emotion* — *body locations* — *resolution*

Relaxation Remembrance
trigger (sticker, red light...) — *working?*

Y N
Y N
Y N
Y N

Mood Check
morning

afternoon

evening

The Relaxation Solution
Daily Journal

Today is _____
M T W T F S S

Theme of the Day

Exercises I Did
time — *duration* — *exercise* — *notes*

Tension I Observed
trigger — *emotion* — *body locations* — *resolution*

Relaxation Remembrance
trigger (sticker, red light...) — *working?*

Y N
Y N
Y N
Y N

Mood Check
morning

afternoon

evening

The Relaxation Solution
Daily Journal

Today is _____
M T W T F S S

Theme of the Day

Exercises I Did
time — *duration* — *exercise* — *notes*

Tension I Observed
trigger — *emotion* — *body locations* — *resolution*

Relaxation Remembrance
trigger (sticker, red light...) — *working?*

Y N
Y N
Y N
Y N

Mood Check

morning

afternoon

evening

The Relaxation Solution

Weekly Journal

Today is _____

M T W T F S S

Theme of the Week

Notes to Self

The Relaxation Solution
Daily Journal

Today is _____
M T W T F S S

Theme of the Day

Exercises I Did
time — *duration* — *exercise* — *notes*

Tension I Observed
trigger — *emotion* — *body locations* — *resolution*

Relaxation Remembrance
trigger (sticker, red light...) — *working?*

Y N
Y N
Y N
Y N

Mood Check
morning

afternoon

evening

The Relaxation Solution
Daily Journal

Today is _____

M T W T F S S

Theme of the Day

Exercises I Did

time — *duration* — *exercise* — *notes*

Tension I Observed

trigger — *emotion* — *body locations* — *resolution*

Relaxation Remembrance

trigger (sticker, red light...) — *working?*

Y   N
Y   N
Y   N
Y   N

Mood Check

morning

😊 😐 🙁 😖 😒 😮

afternoon

😊 😐 🙁 😖 😒 😮

evening

😊 😐 🙁 😖 😒 😮

The Relaxation Solution
Daily Journal

Today is _____

M T W T F S S

Theme of the Day

Exercises I Did
time — duration — exercise — notes

Tension I Observed
trigger — emotion — body locations — resolution

Relaxation Remembrance
trigger (sticker, red light...) — working?

Y N
Y N
Y N
Y N

Mood Check
morning

afternoon

evening

The Relaxation Solution
Daily Journal

Today is _____

M T W T F S S

Theme of the Day

Exercises I Did

time   *duration*   *exercise*   *notes*

Tension I Observed

trigger   *emotion*   *body locations*   *resolution*

Relaxation Remembrance

trigger (sticker, red light...)   *working?*

Y   N
Y   N
Y   N
Y   N

Mood Check

morning

afternoon

evening

The Relaxation Solution
Daily Journal

Today is _____
M T W T F S S

Theme of the Day

Exercises I Did
time — *duration* — *exercise* — *notes*

Tension I Observed
trigger — *emotion* — *body locations* — *resolution*

Relaxation Remembrance
trigger (sticker, red light...) — *working?*

Y N
Y N
Y N
Y N

Mood Check
morning

afternoon

evening

The Relaxation Solution
Daily Journal

Today is _____
M T W T F S S

Theme of the Day

Exercises I Did
time — duration — exercise — notes

Tension I Observed
trigger — emotion — body locations — resolution

Relaxation Remembrance
trigger (sticker, red light...) — working?

Y N
Y N
Y N
Y N

Mood Check
morning

afternoon

evening

The Relaxation Solution
Daily Journal

Today is _____
M T W T F S S

Theme of the Day

Exercises I Did
time *duration* *exercise* *notes*

Tension I Observed
trigger *emotion* *body locations* *resolution*

Relaxation Remembrance
trigger (sticker, red light...) *working?*

Y N
Y N
Y N
Y N

Mood Check
morning

afternoon

evening

The Relaxation Solution

Weekly Journal

Today is _____

M T W T F S S

Theme of the Week

Notes to Self

The Relaxation Solution
Monthly Self-Evaluation

Today is _____

M T W T F S S

Instructions
Thinking about your life during the past month, answer each question honestly. Don't try to add up specific events. Just respond with your impression or estimate. Write your answer in the *raw* column.

Answers
0 – never   1 – rarely   2 – sometimes   3 – often   4 – very often

Questions

answer: — raw — adj

1. How often have you been upset because of something that happened unexpectedly? ___ → ___
2. How often have you felt that you were unable to control the important things in your life? ___ → ___
3. How often have you felt nervous and stressed? ___ → ___
4. How often have you felt confident about your ability to handle your personal problems? ___ 4-↵ ___
5. How often have you felt that things were going your way? ___ 4-↵ ___
6. How often have you found that you could not cope with all the things that you had to do? ___ → ___
7. How often have you been able to control irritations in your life? ___ 4-↵ ___
8. How often have you felt that you were on top of things? ___ 4-↵ ___
9. How often have you been angered because of things that happened outside of your control? ___ → ___
10. How often have you felt difficulties were piling up so high you could not overcome them? ___ → ___

Total: ___

Scoring
Write an adjusted score in the *adj* column. To calculate *adj*:
For questions 4, 5, 7, and 8, subtract raw score from 4
(change 0 to 4, 1 to 3, 2 to 2, 3 to 1, and 4 to 0.)
For questions 1, 2, 3, 6, 9, and 10, copy the raw score into *adj*.

Evaluation
If your total adjusted score is...
0 to 13 - your stress level is **low**.
14 to 26 - your stress level is **moderate**.
27 to 40 - your stress level is **high**.

The Relaxation Solution
Daily Journal

Today is _____

M T W T F S S

Theme of the Day

Exercises I Did

time	duration	exercise	notes

Tension I Observed

trigger	emotion	body locations	resolution

Relaxation Remembrance

trigger (sticker, red light...) — working?

Y N
Y N
Y N
Y N

Mood Check

morning
☺ 😐 🙁 😣 😠 😮

afternoon
☺ 😐 🙁 😣 😠 😮

evening
☺ 😐 🙁 😣 😠 😮

The Relaxation Solution
Daily Journal

Today is _____
M T W T F S S

Theme of the Day

Exercises I Did
time — duration — exercise — notes

Tension I Observed
trigger — emotion — body locations — resolution

Relaxation Remembrance
trigger (sticker, red light...) — working?

Y N
Y N
Y N
Y N

Mood Check
morning
afternoon
evening

The Relaxation Solution
Daily Journal

Today is _____
M T W T F S S

Theme of the Day

Exercises I Did
time — duration — exercise — notes

Tension I Observed
trigger — emotion — body locations — resolution

Relaxation Remembrance
trigger (sticker, red light...) — *working?*

Y N
Y N
Y N
Y N

Mood Check
morning

afternoon

evening

The Relaxation Solution
Daily Journal

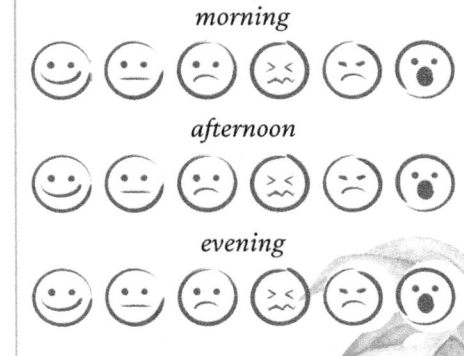

Today is _____
M T W T F S S

Theme of the Day

Exercises I Did
time — *duration* — *exercise* — *notes*

Tension I Observed
trigger — *emotion* — *body locations* — *resolution*

Relaxation Remembrance
trigger (sticker, red light...) — *working?*

Y   N
Y   N
Y   N
Y   N

Mood Check
morning

afternoon

evening

The Relaxation Solution
Daily Journal

Today is _____

M T W T F S S

Theme of the Day

Exercises I Did
time — *duration* — *exercise* — *notes*

Tension I Observed
trigger — *emotion* — *body locations* — *resolution*

Relaxation Remembrance
trigger (sticker, red light...) — *working?*

Y N
Y N
Y N
Y N

Mood Check

morning

afternoon

evening

The Relaxation Solution
Daily Journal

Today is _____
M T W T F S S

Theme of the Day

Exercises I Did
time — *duration* — *exercise* — *notes*

Tension I Observed
trigger — *emotion* — *body locations* — *resolution*

Relaxation Remembrance
trigger (sticker, red light...) — *working?*

Y N
Y N
Y N
Y N

Mood Check
morning

afternoon

evening

The Relaxation Solution
Daily Journal

Today is _____

M T W T F S S

Theme of the Day

Exercises I Did

time	duration	exercise	notes

Tension I Observed

trigger	emotion	body locations	resolution

Relaxation Remembrance

trigger (sticker, red light...)   working?

Y   N
Y   N
Y   N
Y   N

Mood Check

morning

afternoon

evening

The Relaxation Solution

Weekly Journal

Today is _____

M T W T F S S

― Theme of the Week ―

― Notes to Self ―

The Relaxation Solution
Daily Journal

Today is _____

M T W T F S S

Theme of the Day

Exercises I Did
time — duration — exercise — notes

Tension I Observed
trigger — emotion — body locations — resolution

Relaxation Remembrance
trigger (sticker, red light...) — working?

Y N
Y N
Y N
Y N

Mood Check
morning

afternoon

evening

The Relaxation Solution
Daily Journal

Today is _____
M T W T F S S

Theme of the Day

Exercises I Did
time *duration* *exercise* *notes*

Tension I Observed
trigger *emotion* *body locations* *resolution*

Relaxation Remembrance
trigger (sticker, red light...) *working?*

Y N
Y N
Y N
Y N

Mood Check
morning

afternoon

evening

The Relaxation Solution
Daily Journal

Today is _____
M T W T F S S

Theme of the Day

Exercises I Did
time — duration — exercise — notes

Tension I Observed
trigger — emotion — body locations — resolution

Relaxation Remembrance
trigger (sticker, red light...) — working?

Y N
Y N
Y N
Y N

Mood Check
morning

afternoon

evening

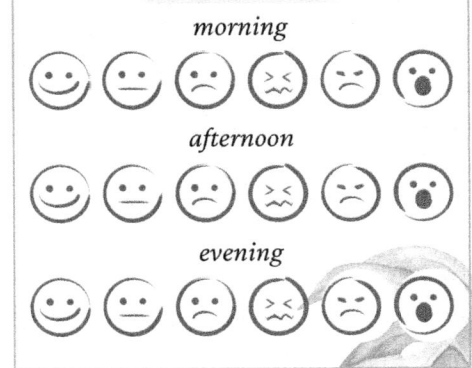

The Relaxation Solution
Daily Journal

Today is _____
M T W T F S S

Theme of the Day

Exercises I Did
time — *duration* — *exercise* — *notes*

Tension I Observed
trigger — *emotion* — *body locations* — *resolution*

Relaxation Remembrance
trigger (sticker, red light...) — *working?*

Y N
Y N
Y N
Y N

Mood Check
morning

afternoon

evening

The Relaxation Solution
Daily Journal

Today is _____

M T W T F S S

Theme of the Day

Exercises I Did
time — *duration* — *exercise* — *notes*

Tension I Observed
trigger — *emotion* — *body locations* — *resolution*

Relaxation Remembrance
trigger (sticker, red light...) — *working?*

Y N
Y N
Y N
Y N

Mood Check
morning

afternoon

evening

The Relaxation Solution
Daily Journal

Today is _____
M T W T F S S

Theme of the Day

Exercises I Did
time — *duration* — *exercise* — *notes*

Tension I Observed
trigger — *emotion* — *body locations* — *resolution*

Relaxation Remembrance
trigger (sticker, red light...) — *working?*

Y N
Y N
Y N
Y N

Mood Check
morning

afternoon

evening

The Relaxation Solution
Daily Journal

Today is _____
M T W T F S S

Theme of the Day

Exercises I Did
time — *duration* — *exercise* — *notes*

Tension I Observed
trigger — *emotion* — *body locations* — *resolution*

Relaxation Remembrance
trigger (sticker, red light...) — *working?*

Y N
Y N
Y N
Y N

Mood Check
morning

afternoon

evening

The Relaxation Solution

Weekly Journal

Today is _____
M T W T F S S

Theme of the Week

Notes to Self

The Relaxation Solution
Daily Journal

Today is _____
M T W T F S S

Theme of the Day

Exercises I Did
— time — duration — exercise — notes

Tension I Observed
— trigger — emotion — body locations — resolution

Relaxation Remembrance
— trigger (sticker, red light...) — working?

Y N
Y N
Y N
Y N

Mood Check
morning
afternoon
evening

The Relaxation Solution
Daily Journal

Today is _____
M T W T F S S

Theme of the Day

Exercises I Did
time — *duration* — *exercise* — *notes*

Tension I Observed
trigger — *emotion* — *body locations* — *resolution*

Relaxation Remembrance
trigger (sticker, red light...) — *working?*

Y N
Y N
Y N
Y N

Mood Check
morning

afternoon

evening

The Relaxation Solution
Daily Journal

Today is _____
M T W T F S S

Theme of the Day

Exercises I Did
time — *duration* — *exercise* — *notes*

Tension I Observed
trigger — *emotion* — *body locations* — *resolution*

Relaxation Remembrance
trigger (sticker, red light...) — *working?*

Y N
Y N
Y N
Y N

Mood Check

morning
😊 😐 ☹️ 😣 😒 😮

afternoon
😊 😐 ☹️ 😣 😒 😮

evening
😊 😐 ☹️ 😣 😒 😮

The Relaxation Solution
Daily Journal

Today is _____
M T W T F S S

Theme of the Day

Exercises I Did
time — *duration* — *exercise* — *notes*

Tension I Observed
trigger — *emotion* — *body locations* — *resolution*

Relaxation Remembrance
trigger (sticker, red light...) — *working?*

Y   N
Y   N
Y   N
Y   N

Mood Check
morning

afternoon

evening

The Relaxation Solution
Daily Journal

Today is _____

M T W T F S S

Theme of the Day

Exercises I Did
time — *duration* — *exercise* — *notes*

Tension I Observed
trigger — *emotion* — *body locations* — *resolution*

Relaxation Remembrance
trigger (sticker, red light...) — *working?*

Y N
Y N
Y N
Y N

Mood Check
morning

afternoon

evening

The Relaxation Solution
Daily Journal

Today is _____
M T W T F S S

Theme of the Day

Exercises I Did
time — *duration* — *exercise* — *notes*

Tension I Observed
trigger — *emotion* — *body locations* — *resolution*

Relaxation Remembrance
trigger (sticker, red light...) — *working?*

Y N
Y N
Y N
Y N

Mood Check
morning

afternoon

evening

The Relaxation Solution
Daily Journal

Today is _____

M T W T F S S

Theme of the Day

Exercises I Did
time — *duration* — *exercise* — *notes*

Tension I Observed
trigger — *emotion* — *body locations* — *resolution*

Relaxation Remembrance
trigger (sticker, red light...) — *working?*

Y N
Y N
Y N
Y N

Mood Check
morning

afternoon

evening

The Relaxation Solution
Weekly Journal

Today is _____
M T W T F S S

Theme of the Week

Notes to Self

The Relaxation Solution

Daily Journal

Today is _____

M T W T F S S

Theme of the Day

Exercises I Did

time	duration	exercise	notes

Tension I Observed

trigger	emotion	body locations	resolution

Relaxation Remembrance

trigger (sticker, red light...)	working?
	Y N
	Y N
	Y N
	Y N

Mood Check

morning

😊 😐 🙁 😖 😒 😮

afternoon

😊 😐 🙁 😖 😒 😮

evening

😊 😐 🙁 😖 😒 😮

The Relaxation Solution
Daily Journal

Today is _____
M T W T F S S

Theme of the Day

Exercises I Did
time — *duration* — *exercise* — *notes*

Tension I Observed
trigger — *emotion* — *body locations* — *resolution*

Relaxation Remembrance
trigger (sticker, red light...) — *working?*

Y N
Y N
Y N
Y N

Mood Check
morning
afternoon
evening

The Relaxation Solution
Daily Journal

Today is _____

M T W T F S S

Theme of the Day

Exercises I Did
time — *duration* — *exercise* — *notes*

Tension I Observed
trigger — *emotion* — *body locations* — *resolution*

Relaxation Remembrance
trigger (sticker, red light...) — working?

Y N
Y N
Y N
Y N

Mood Check
morning

afternoon

evening

The Relaxation Solution
Daily Journal

Today is _____
M T W T F S S

Theme of the Day

Exercises I Did
time — *duration* — *exercise* — *notes*

Tension I Observed
trigger — *emotion* — *body locations* — *resolution*

Relaxation Remembrance
trigger (sticker, red light...) — *working?*

Y N
Y N
Y N
Y N

Mood Check
morning

afternoon

evening

The Relaxation Solution
Daily Journal

Today is _____
M T W T F S S

Theme of the Day

Exercises I Did
time — *duration* — *exercise* — *notes*

Tension I Observed
trigger — *emotion* — *body locations* — *resolution*

Relaxation Remembrance
trigger (sticker, red light...) — *working?*

Y N
Y N
Y N
Y N

Mood Check
morning
😊 😐 🙁 😖 😒 😮

afternoon
😊 😐 🙁 😖 😒 😮

evening
😊 😐 🙁 😖 😒 😮

The Relaxation Solution
Daily Journal

Today is _____
M T W T F S S

Theme of the Day

Exercises I Did
time — *duration* — *exercise* — *notes*

Tension I Observed
trigger — *emotion* — *body locations* — *resolution*

Relaxation Remembrance
trigger (sticker, red light...) — *working?*

Y   N
Y   N
Y   N
Y   N

Mood Check
morning

afternoon

evening

The Relaxation Solution
Daily Journal

Today is _____

M T W T F S S

Theme of the Day

Exercises I Did
time — duration — exercise — notes

Tension I Observed
trigger — emotion — body locations — resolution

Relaxation Remembrance
trigger (sticker, red light...) — working?

Y N
Y N
Y N
Y N

Mood Check
morning

afternoon

evening

The Relaxation Solution

Weekly Journal

Today is _____

M T W T F S S

Theme of the Week

Notes to Self

The Relaxation Solution
Monthly Self-Evaluation

Today is _____
M T W T F S S

Instructions
Thinking about your life during the past month, answer each question honestly. Don't try to add up specific events. Just respond with your impression or estimate. Write your answer in the *raw* column.

Answers
0 – never   1 – rarely   2 – sometimes   3 – often   4 – very often

Questions

answer: — raw — adj

1. How often have you been upset because of something that happened unexpectedly? →
2. How often have you felt that you were unable to control the important things in your life? →
3. How often have you felt nervous and stressed? →
4. How often have you felt confident about your ability to handle your personal problems? 4-
5. How often have you felt that things were going your way? 4-
6. How often have you found that you could not cope with all the things that you had to do? →
7. How often have you been able to control irritations in your life? 4-
8. How often have you felt that you were on top of things? 4-
9. How often have you been angered because of things that happened outside of your control? →
10. How often have you felt difficulties were piling up so high you could not overcome them? →

Total: ____

Scoring
Write an adjusted score in the *adj* column. To calculate *adj*:
For questions 4, 5, 7, and 8, subtract raw score from 4
(change 0 to 4, 1 to 3, 2 to 2, 3 to 1, and 4 to 0.)
For questions 1, 2, 3, 6, 9, and 10, copy the raw score into *adj*.

Evaluation
If your total adjusted score is...

0 to 13 - your stress level is **low**.
14 to 26 - your stress level is **moderate**.
27 to 40 - your stress level is **high**.

The Relaxation Solution
Daily Journal

Today is _____
M T W T F S S

Theme of the Day

Exercises I Did
time — *duration* — *exercise* — *notes*

Tension I Observed
trigger — *emotion* — *body locations* — *resolution*

Relaxation Remembrance
trigger (sticker, red light...) — *working?*

Y N
Y N
Y N
Y N

Mood Check
morning

afternoon

evening

The Relaxation Solution
Daily Journal

Today is _____

M T W T F S S

Theme of the Day

Exercises I Did
time — duration — exercise — notes

Tension I Observed
trigger — emotion — body locations — resolution

Relaxation Remembrance
trigger (sticker, red light...) — working?

Y N
Y N
Y N
Y N

Mood Check

morning

afternoon

evening

The Relaxation Solution
Daily Journal

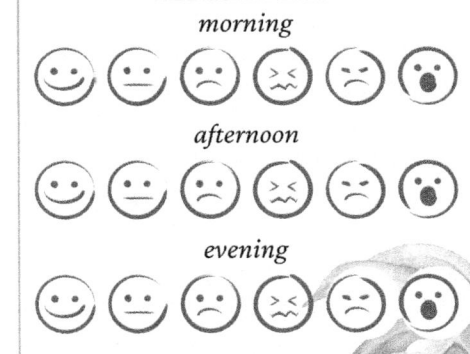

Today is _____
M T W T F S S

Theme of the Day

Exercises I Did
time — *duration* — *exercise* — *notes*

Tension I Observed
trigger — *emotion* — *body locations* — *resolution*

Relaxation Remembrance
trigger (sticker, red light...) — *working?*

Y N
Y N
Y N
Y N

Mood Check
morning

afternoon

evening

The Relaxation Solution
Daily Journal

Today is _____

M T W T F S S

Theme of the Day

Exercises I Did
time — *duration* — *exercise* — *notes*

Tension I Observed
trigger — *emotion* — *body locations* — *resolution*

Relaxation Remembrance
trigger (sticker, red light...) — *working?*

Y N
Y N
Y N
Y N

Mood Check
morning

afternoon

evening

The Relaxation Solution
Daily Journal

Today is _____
M T W T F S S

Theme of the Day

Exercises I Did
time — *duration* — *exercise* — *notes*

Tension I Observed
trigger — *emotion* — *body locations* — *resolution*

Relaxation Remembrance
trigger (sticker, red light...) — *working?*

Y N
Y N
Y N
Y N

Mood Check
morning

afternoon

evening

The Relaxation Solution
Daily Journal

Today is _____

M T W T F S S

Theme of the Day

Exercises I Did
time — duration — exercise — notes

Tension I Observed
trigger — emotion — body locations — resolution

Relaxation Remembrance
trigger (sticker, red light...) — *working?*

Y N
Y N
Y N
Y N

Mood Check
morning
😊 😐 ☹️ 😣 😒 😮

afternoon
😊 😐 ☹️ 😣 😒 😮

evening
😊 😐 ☹️ 😣 😒 😮

The Relaxation Solution
Daily Journal

Today is _____
M T W T F S S

Theme of the Day

Exercises I Did
time — *duration* — *exercise* — *notes*

Tension I Observed
trigger — *emotion* — *body locations* — *resolution*

Relaxation Remembrance
trigger (sticker, red light...) — *working?*

Y N
Y N
Y N
Y N

Mood Check
morning

afternoon

evening

The Relaxation Solution
Weekly Journal

Today is _____

M T W T F S S

Theme of the Week

Notes to Self

The Relaxation Solution
Daily Journal

Today is _____

M T W T F S S

Theme of the Day

Exercises I Did
time — *duration* — *exercise* — *notes*

Tension I Observed
trigger — *emotion* — *body locations* — *resolution*

Relaxation Remembrance
trigger (sticker, red light...) — *working?*

Y N
Y N
Y N
Y N

Mood Check
morning
😊 😐 🙁 😣 😠 😮

afternoon
😊 😐 🙁 😣 😠 😮

evening
😊 😐 🙁 😣 😠 😮

The Relaxation Solution
Daily Journal

Today is _____

M T W T F S S

Theme of the Day

Exercises I Did
time — *duration* — *exercise* — *notes*

Tension I Observed
trigger — *emotion* — *body locations* — *resolution*

Relaxation Remembrance
trigger (sticker, red light...) — *working?*

Y N
Y N
Y N
Y N

Mood Check
morning

afternoon

evening

The Relaxation Solution
Daily Journal

Today is _____
M T W T F S S

Theme of the Day

Exercises I Did
time — duration — exercise — notes

Tension I Observed
trigger — emotion — body locations — resolution

Relaxation Remembrance
trigger (sticker, red light...) — working?

Y N
Y N
Y N
Y N

Mood Check
morning

afternoon

evening

The Relaxation Solution

Daily Journal

Today is _____

M T W T F S S

Theme of the Day

Exercises I Did

time — *duration* — *exercise* — *notes*

Tension I Observed

trigger — *emotion* — *body locations* — *resolution*

Relaxation Remembrance

trigger (sticker, red light...) — *working?*

Y   N
Y   N
Y   N
Y   N

Mood Check

morning

afternoon

evening

The Relaxation Solution
Daily Journal

Today is _____
M T W T F S S

Theme of the Day

Exercises I Did
time — duration — exercise — notes

Tension I Observed
trigger — emotion — body locations — resolution

Relaxation Remembrance
trigger (sticker, red light...) — *working?*

Y N
Y N
Y N
Y N

Mood Check
morning

afternoon

evening

The Relaxation Solution
Daily Journal

Today is _____
M T W T F S S

Theme of the Day

Exercises I Did
time — *duration* — *exercise* — *notes*

Tension I Observed
trigger — *emotion* — *body locations* — *resolution*

Relaxation Remembrance
trigger (sticker, red light…) — *working?*

Y   N
Y   N
Y   N
Y   N

Mood Check
morning

afternoon

evening

The Relaxation Solution
Daily Journal

Today is _____
M T W T F S S

Theme of the Day

Exercises I Did
time — *duration* — *exercise* — *notes*

Tension I Observed
trigger — *emotion* — *body locations* — *resolution*

Relaxation Remembrance
trigger (sticker, red light...) — *working?*

Y N
Y N
Y N
Y N

Mood Check
morning

afternoon

evening

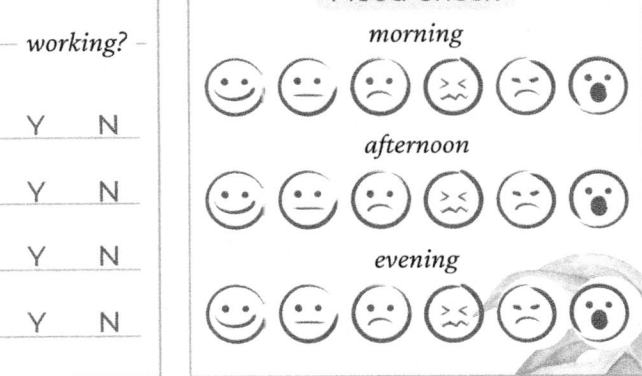

The Relaxation Solution

Weekly Journal

Today is _____

M T W T F S S

Theme of the Week

Notes to Self

The Relaxation Solution
Daily Journal

Today is _____
M T W T F S S

Theme of the Day

Exercises I Did
time   *duration*   *exercise*   *notes*

Tension I Observed
trigger   *emotion*   *body locations*   *resolution*

Relaxation Remembrance
trigger (sticker, red light...)   *working?*

Y N
Y N
Y N
Y N

Mood Check
morning

afternoon

evening

The Relaxation Solution
Daily Journal

Today is _____
M T W T F S S

Theme of the Day

Exercises I Did
time — *duration* — *exercise* — *notes*

Tension I Observed
trigger — *emotion* — *body locations* — *resolution*

Relaxation Remembrance
trigger (sticker, red light...) — *working?*

Y   N
Y   N
Y   N
Y   N

Mood Check
morning

afternoon

evening

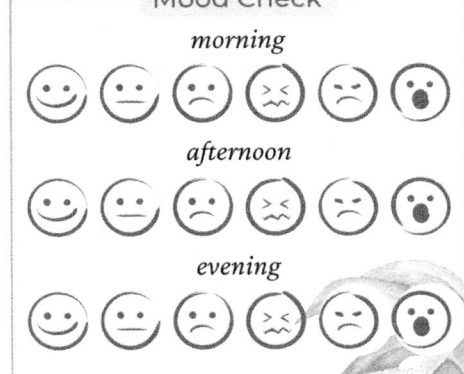

The Relaxation Solution
Daily Journal

Today is _____
M T W T F S S

Theme of the Day

Exercises I Did
time — *duration* — *exercise* — *notes*

Tension I Observed
trigger — *emotion* — *body locations* — *resolution*

Relaxation Remembrance
trigger (sticker, red light...) — *working?*

Y N
Y N
Y N
Y N

Mood Check
morning
afternoon
evening

The Relaxation Solution
Daily Journal

Today is _____
M T W T F S S

Theme of the Day

Exercises I Did
time — duration — exercise — notes

Tension I Observed
trigger — emotion — body locations — resolution

Relaxation Remembrance
trigger (sticker, red light...) — *working?*

- Y N
- Y N
- Y N
- Y N

Mood Check
morning

afternoon

evening

The Relaxation Solution
Daily Journal

Today is _____
M T W T F S S

Theme of the Day

Exercises I Did
time — *duration* — *exercise* — *notes*

Tension I Observed
trigger — *emotion* — *body locations* — *resolution*

Relaxation Remembrance
trigger (sticker, red light...) — *working?*

Y N
Y N
Y N
Y N

Mood Check
morning

afternoon

evening

The Relaxation Solution
Daily Journal

Today is ____
M T W T F S S

Theme of the Day

Exercises I Did
time — duration — exercise — notes

Tension I Observed
trigger — emotion — body locations — resolution

Relaxation Remembrance
trigger (sticker, red light...) — working?

Y N
Y N
Y N
Y N

Mood Check
morning

afternoon

evening

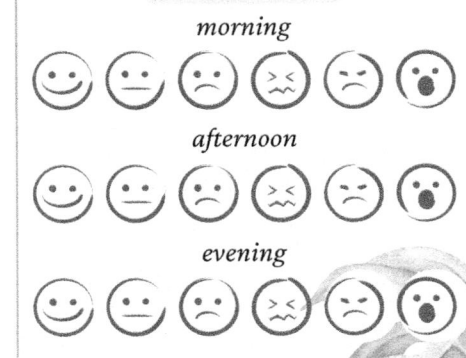

The Relaxation Solution
Daily Journal

Today is _____
M T W T F S S

Theme of the Day

Exercises I Did
time — duration — exercise — notes

Tension I Observed
trigger — emotion — body locations — resolution

Relaxation Remembrance
trigger (sticker, red light...) — working?

Y N
Y N
Y N
Y N

Mood Check
morning
afternoon
evening

The Relaxation Solution

Weekly Journal

Today is _____

M T W T F S S

Theme of the Week

Notes to Self

The Relaxation Solution
Daily Journal

Today is _____
M T W T F S S

Theme of the Day

Exercises I Did
time — duration — exercise — notes

Tension I Observed
trigger — emotion — body locations — resolution

Relaxation Remembrance
trigger (sticker, red light...) — working?

Y   N
Y   N
Y   N
Y   N

Mood Check
morning
😊 😐 🙁 😖 😠 😮

afternoon
😊 😐 🙁 😖 😠 😮

evening
😊 😐 🙁 😖 😠 😮

The Relaxation Solution
Daily Journal

Today is _____
M T W T F S S

Theme of the Day

Exercises I Did
time   *duration*   *exercise*   *notes*

Tension I Observed
trigger   *emotion*   *body locations*   *resolution*

Relaxation Remembrance
trigger (sticker, red light...)   *working?*

Y N
Y N
Y N
Y N

Mood Check
morning

afternoon

evening

The Relaxation Solution
Daily Journal

Today is _____
M T W T F S S

Theme of the Day

Exercises I Did
time — duration — exercise — notes

Tension I Observed
trigger — emotion — body locations — resolution

Relaxation Remembrance
trigger (sticker, red light...) — working?

Y N
Y N
Y N
Y N

Mood Check
morning

afternoon

evening

The Relaxation Solution
Daily Journal

Today is _____
M T W T F S S

Theme of the Day

Exercises I Did
time — duration — exercise — notes

Tension I Observed
trigger — emotion — body locations — resolution

Relaxation Remembrance
trigger (sticker, red light...) — working?

Y N
Y N
Y N
Y N

Mood Check
morning

afternoon

evening

The Relaxation Solution
Daily Journal

Today is _____
M T W T F S S

Theme of the Day

Exercises I Did
time — *duration* — *exercise* — *notes*

Tension I Observed
trigger — *emotion* — *body locations* — *resolution*

Relaxation Remembrance
trigger (sticker, red light...) — *working?*

Y N
Y N
Y N
Y N

Mood Check
morning

afternoon

evening

The Relaxation Solution
Daily Journal

Today is _____

M T W T F S S

Theme of the Day

Exercises I Did
time — *duration* — *exercise* — *notes*

Tension I Observed
trigger — *emotion* — *body locations* — *resolution*

Relaxation Remembrance
trigger (sticker, red light...) — *working?*

Y N
Y N
Y N
Y N

Mood Check
morning

afternoon

evening

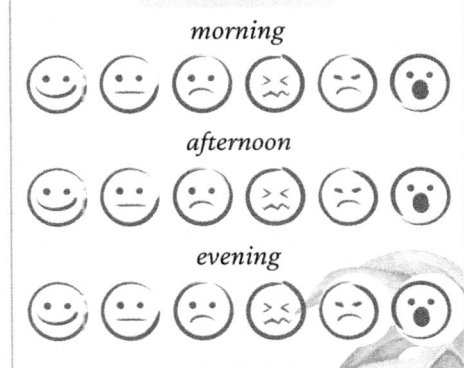

The Relaxation Solution
Daily Journal

Today is _____
M T W T F S S

Theme of the Day

Exercises I Did
time — duration — exercise — notes

Tension I Observed
trigger — emotion — body locations — resolution

Relaxation Remembrance
trigger (sticker, red light...) — working?

Y N
Y N
Y N
Y N

Mood Check
morning

afternoon

evening

The Relaxation Solution

Weekly Journal

Today is _____

M T W T F S S

Theme of the Week

Notes to Self

The Relaxation Solution
Monthly Self-Evaluation

Today is _____

M T W T F S S

Instructions

Thinking about your life during the past month, answer each question honestly. Don't try to add up specific events. Just respond with your impression or estimate. Write your answer in the *raw* column.

Answers

0 – never   1 – rarely   2 – sometimes   3 – often   4 – very often

Questions

answer: — raw — adj

1. How often have you been upset because of something that happened unexpectedly? ___ → ___

2. How often have you felt that you were unable to control the important things in your life? ___ → ___

3. How often have you felt nervous and stressed? ___ → ___

4. How often have you felt confident about your ability to handle your personal problems? ___ 4-↘ ___

5. How often have you felt that things were going your way? ___ 4-↘ ___

6. How often have you found that you could not cope with all the things that you had to do? ___ → ___

7. How often have you been able to control irritations in your life? ___ 4-↘ ___

8. How often have you felt that you were on top of things? ___ 4-↘ ___

9. How often have you been angered because of things that happened outside of your control? ___ → ___

10. How often have you felt difficulties were piling up so high you could not overcome them? ___ → ___

Total: ___

Scoring

Write an adjusted score in the *adj* column. To calculate *adj*:
For questions 4, 5, 7, and 8, subtract raw score from 4
(change 0 to 4, 1 to 3, 2 to 2, 3 to 1, and 4 to 0.)
For questions 1, 2, 3, 6, 9, and 10, copy the raw score into *adj*.

Evaluation

If your total adjusted score is...

0 to 13 - your stress level is **low**.
14 to 26 - your stress level is **moderate**.
27 to 40 - your stress level is **high**.

The Relaxation Solution
Daily Journal

Today is _____
M T W T F S S

Theme of the Day

Exercises I Did
time — duration — exercise — notes

Tension I Observed
trigger — emotion — body locations — resolution

Relaxation Remembrance
trigger (sticker, red light...) — working?

Y N
Y N
Y N
Y N

Mood Check
morning

afternoon

evening

The Relaxation Solution
Daily Journal

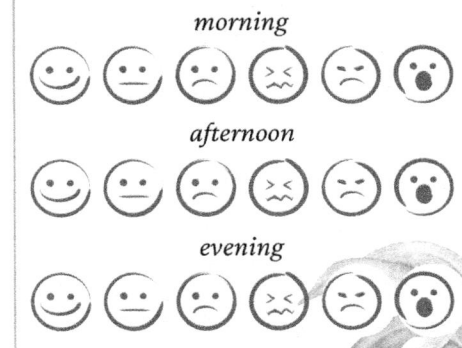

Today is _____
M T W T F S S

Theme of the Day

Exercises I Did
time — *duration* — *exercise* — *notes*

Tension I Observed
trigger — *emotion* — *body locations* — *resolution*

Relaxation Remembrance
trigger (sticker, red light...) — *working?*

Y N
Y N
Y N
Y N

Mood Check
morning

afternoon

evening

The Relaxation Solution
Daily Journal

Today is _____
M T W T F S S

Theme of the Day

Exercises I Did
time — duration — exercise — notes

Tension I Observed
trigger — emotion — body locations — resolution

Relaxation Remembrance
trigger (sticker, red light...) — working?

Y N
Y N
Y N
Y N

Mood Check
morning
😊 😐 🙁 😣 😠 😮

afternoon
😊 😐 🙁 😣 😠 😮

evening
😊 😐 🙁 😣 😠 😮

The Relaxation Solution
Daily Journal

Today is _____
M T W T F S S

Theme of the Day

Exercises I Did
time — *duration* — *exercise* — *notes*

Tension I Observed
trigger — *emotion* — *body locations* — *resolution*

Relaxation Remembrance
trigger (sticker, red light...) — *working?*

Y N
Y N
Y N
Y N

Mood Check
morning
afternoon
evening

The Relaxation Solution
Daily Journal

Today is _____

M T W T F S S

Theme of the Day

Exercises I Did
— time — duration — exercise — notes —

Tension I Observed
— trigger — emotion — body locations — resolution —

Relaxation Remembrance
— trigger (sticker, red light...) — working? —

Y N
Y N
Y N
Y N

Mood Check
morning
😊 😐 🙁 😖 😒 😮

afternoon
😊 😐 🙁 😖 😒 😮

evening
😊 😐 🙁 😖 😒 😮

The Relaxation Solution
Daily Journal

Today is _____
M T W T F S S

Theme of the Day

Exercises I Did
time — *duration* — *exercise* — *notes*

Tension I Observed
trigger — *emotion* — *body locations* — *resolution*

Relaxation Remembrance
trigger (sticker, red light...) — *working?*

Y N
Y N
Y N
Y N

Mood Check
morning
afternoon
evening

The Relaxation Solution

Daily Journal

Today is _____
M T W T F S S

Theme of the Day

Exercises I Did
time — duration — exercise — notes

Tension I Observed
trigger — emotion — body locations — resolution

Relaxation Remembrance
trigger (sticker, red light...) — *working?*

Y N
Y N
Y N
Y N

Mood Check

morning
😊 😐 🙁 😣 😒 😮

afternoon
😊 😐 🙁 😣 😒 😮

evening
😊 😐 🙁 😣 😒 😮

The Relaxation Solution

— Weekly Journal —

Today is _____

M T W T F S S

— Theme of the Week —

— Notes to Self —

The Relaxation Solution
Daily Journal

Today is _____
M T W T F S S

Theme of the Day

Exercises I Did
time — *duration* — *exercise* — *notes*

Tension I Observed
trigger — *emotion* — *body locations* — *resolution*

Relaxation Remembrance
trigger (sticker, red light...) — *working?*

Y N
Y N
Y N
Y N

Mood Check
morning
afternoon
evening

The Relaxation Solution
Daily Journal

Today is _____
M T W T F S S

Theme of the Day

Exercises I Did
time — *duration* — *exercise* — *notes*

Tension I Observed
trigger — *emotion* — *body locations* — *resolution*

Relaxation Remembrance
trigger (sticker, red light...) — working?

Y N
Y N
Y N
Y N

Mood Check
morning

afternoon

evening

The Relaxation Solution

Daily Journal

Today is _____
M T W T F S S

Theme of the Day

Exercises I Did
time — duration — exercise — notes

Tension I Observed
trigger — emotion — body locations — resolution

Relaxation Remembrance
trigger (sticker, red light...) — working?

Y N
Y N
Y N
Y N

Mood Check
morning

afternoon

evening

The Relaxation Solution
Daily Journal

Today is _____
M T W T F S S

Theme of the Day

Exercises I Did
time *duration* *exercise* *notes*

Tension I Observed
trigger *emotion* *body locations* *resolution*

Relaxation Remembrance
trigger (sticker, red light…) *working?*

Y N
Y N
Y N
Y N

Mood Check
morning
afternoon
evening

The Relaxation Solution
Daily Journal

Today is _____
M T W T F S S

Theme of the Day

Exercises I Did
time — *duration* — *exercise* — *notes*

Tension I Observed
trigger — *emotion* — *body locations* — *resolution*

Relaxation Remembrance
trigger (sticker, red light...) — *working?*

Y N
Y N
Y N
Y N

Mood Check
morning
afternoon
evening

The Relaxation Solution
Daily Journal

Today is _____
M T W T F S S

Theme of the Day

Exercises I Did
— time — duration — exercise — notes

Tension I Observed
— trigger — emotion — body locations — resolution

Relaxation Remembrance
— trigger (sticker, red light...) — working?

Y N
Y N
Y N
Y N

Mood Check
morning

afternoon

evening

The Relaxation Solution
Daily Journal

Today is _____
M T W T F S S

Theme of the Day

Exercises I Did
time — duration — exercise — notes

Tension I Observed
trigger — emotion — body locations — resolution

Relaxation Remembrance
trigger (sticker, red light...) — working?

Y N
Y N
Y N
Y N

Mood Check
morning
😊 😐 🙁 😣 😠 😮

afternoon
😊 😐 🙁 😣 😠 😮

evening
😊 😐 🙁 😣 😠 😮

The Relaxation Solution

Weekly Journal

Today is _____

M T W T F S S

Theme of the Week

Notes to Self

The Relaxation Solution
Daily Journal

Today is _____
M T W T F S S

Theme of the Day

Exercises I Did
time — duration — exercise — notes

Tension I Observed
trigger — emotion — body locations — resolution

Relaxation Remembrance
trigger (sticker, red light...) — working?

Y N
Y N
Y N
Y N

Mood Check
morning
😊 😐 🙁 😣 😒 😮

afternoon
😊 😐 🙁 😣 😒 😮

evening
😊 😐 🙁 😣 😒 😮

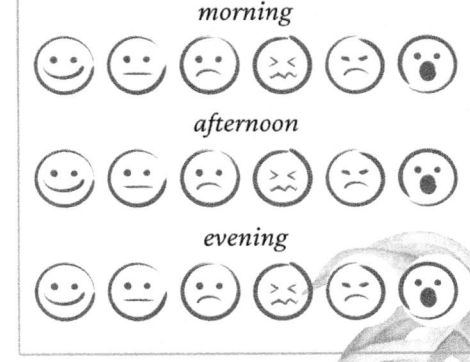

The Relaxation Solution
Daily Journal

Today is _____

M T W T F S S

Theme of the Day

Exercises I Did
time — *duration* — *exercise* — *notes*

Tension I Observed
trigger — *emotion* — *body locations* — *resolution*

Relaxation Remembrance
trigger (sticker, red light...) — *working?*

Y N
Y N
Y N
Y N

Mood Check
morning
afternoon
evening

The Relaxation Solution
Daily Journal

Today is _____

M T W T F S S

Theme of the Day

Exercises I Did
time — duration — exercise — notes

Tension I Observed
trigger — emotion — body locations — resolution

Relaxation Remembrance
trigger (sticker, red light...) — *working?*

Y N
Y N
Y N
Y N

Mood Check
morning
afternoon
evening

The Relaxation Solution
Daily Journal

Today is _____
M T W T F S S

Theme of the Day

Exercises I Did
time — duration — exercise — notes

Tension I Observed
trigger — emotion — body locations — resolution

Relaxation Remembrance
trigger (sticker, red light...) — working?
Y N
Y N
Y N
Y N

Mood Check
morning

afternoon

evening

The Relaxation Solution
Daily Journal

Today is _____

M T W T F S S

Theme of the Day

Exercises I Did
time — *duration* — *exercise* — *notes*

Tension I Observed
trigger — *emotion* — *body locations* — *resolution*

Relaxation Remembrance
trigger (sticker, red light...) — *working?*

Y N
Y N
Y N
Y N

Mood Check
morning
afternoon
evening

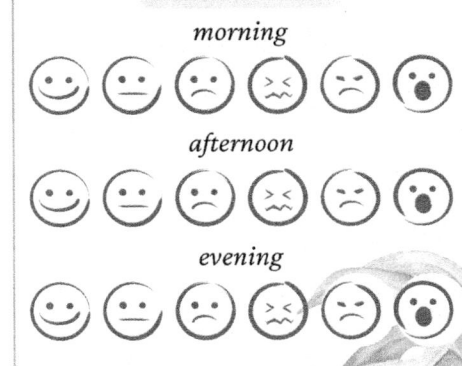

The Relaxation Solution
Daily Journal

Today is _____
M T W T F S S

Theme of the Day

Exercises I Did
— time —— duration —— exercise —————————— notes —

Tension I Observed
— trigger ————— emotion ————— body locations ————— resolution —

Relaxation Remembrance
— trigger (sticker, red light...) ———————— working? —

Y N
Y N
Y N
Y N

Mood Check
morning

afternoon

evening

The Relaxation Solution
Daily Journal

Today is _____
M T W T F S S

Theme of the Day

Exercises I Did
time — duration — exercise — notes

Tension I Observed
trigger — emotion — body locations — resolution

Relaxation Remembrance
trigger (sticker, red light...) — working?

Y N
Y N
Y N
Y N

Mood Check
morning

afternoon

evening

The Relaxation Solution

Weekly Journal

Today is _____

M T W T F S S

Theme of the Week

Notes to Self

The Relaxation Solution
Daily Journal

Today is _____
M T W T F S S

Theme of the Day

Exercises I Did
time — *duration* — *exercise* — *notes*

Tension I Observed
trigger — *emotion* — *body locations* — *resolution*

Relaxation Remembrance
trigger (sticker, red light...) — *working?*

Y   N
Y   N
Y   N
Y   N

Mood Check
morning

afternoon

evening

The Relaxation Solution
Daily Journal

Today is _____
M T W T F S S

Theme of the Day

Exercises I Did
time — duration — exercise — notes

Tension I Observed
trigger — emotion — body locations — resolution

Relaxation Remembrance
trigger (sticker, red light...) — working?

Y N
Y N
Y N
Y N

Mood Check
morning

afternoon

evening

The Relaxation Solution
Daily Journal

Today is _____

M T W T F S S

Theme of the Day

Exercises I Did
time — *duration* — *exercise* — *notes*

Tension I Observed
trigger — *emotion* — *body locations* — *resolution*

Relaxation Remembrance
trigger (sticker, red light...) — *working?*

- Y N
- Y N
- Y N
- Y N

Mood Check
morning
😊 😐 🙁 😖 😠 😮

afternoon
😊 😐 🙁 😖 😠 😮

evening
😊 😐 🙁 😖 😠 😮

The Relaxation Solution
Daily Journal

Today is _____
M T W T F S S

Theme of the Day

Exercises I Did
time — *duration* — *exercise* — *notes*

Tension I Observed
trigger — *emotion* — *body locations* — *resolution*

Relaxation Remembrance
trigger (sticker, red light...) — *working?*

Y N
Y N
Y N
Y N

Mood Check
morning

afternoon

evening

The Relaxation Solution
Daily Journal

Today is _____

M T W T F S S

Theme of the Day

Exercises I Did
time — duration — exercise — notes

Tension I Observed
trigger — emotion — body locations — resolution

Relaxation Remembrance
trigger (sticker, red light...) — working?

Y N
Y N
Y N
Y N

Mood Check
morning

afternoon

evening

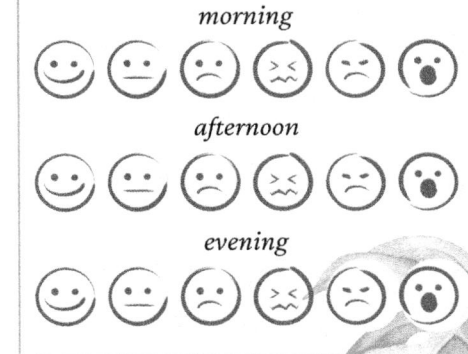

The Relaxation Solution
Daily Journal

Today is _____
M T W T F S S

Theme of the Day

Exercises I Did
time *duration* *exercise* *notes*

Tension I Observed
trigger *emotion* *body locations* *resolution*

Relaxation Remembrance
trigger (sticker, red light...) *working?*

Y N
Y N
Y N
Y N

Mood Check
morning

afternoon

evening

The Relaxation Solution
Daily Journal

Today is _____
M T W T F S S

Theme of the Day

Exercises I Did

time — *duration* — *exercise* — *notes*

Tension I Observed

trigger — *emotion* — *body locations* — *resolution*

Relaxation Remembrance

trigger (sticker, red light...) — *working?*

Y N
Y N
Y N
Y N

Mood Check

morning

afternoon

evening

The Relaxation Solution

Weekly Journal

Today is _____

M T W T F S S

Theme of the Week

Notes to Self

The Relaxation Solution
Monthly Self-Evaluation

Today is _____

M T W T F S S

Instructions

Thinking about your life during the past month, answer each question honestly. Don't try to add up specific events. Just respond with your impression or estimate. Write your answer in the *raw* column.

Answers

0 – never   1 – rarely   2 – sometimes   3 – often   4 – very often

Questions

answer: ——— raw ——— adj

1. How often have you been upset because of something that happened unexpectedly? ___ → ___
2. How often have you felt that you were unable to control the important things in your life? ___ → ___
3. How often have you felt nervous and stressed? ___ → ___
4. How often have you felt confident about your ability to handle your personal problems? ___ 4-↝ ___
5. How often have you felt that things were going your way? ___ 4-↝ ___
6. How often have you found that you could not cope with all the things that you had to do? ___ → ___
7. How often have you been able to control irritations in your life? ___ 4-↝ ___
8. How often have you felt that you were on top of things? ___ 4-↝ ___
9. How often have you been angered because of things that happened outside of your control? ___ → ___
10. How often have you felt difficulties were piling up so high you could not overcome them? ___ → ___

Total: ___

Scoring

Write an adjusted score in the *adj* column. To calculate *adj*:
For questions 4, 5, 7, and 8, subtract raw score from 4
(change 0 to 4, 1 to 3, 2 to 2, 3 to 1, and 4 to 0.)
For questions 1, 2, 3, 6, 9, and 10, copy the raw score into *adj*.

Evaluation

If your total adjusted score is...

0 to 13 - your stress level is **low**.
14 to 26 - your stress level is **moderate**.
27 to 40 - your stress level is **high**.

The Relaxation Solution Workbook and Journal

Was This Book Helpful?

If you have found value here, may I ask a small favor? If you could take a few moments to leave a short review on your favorite online retailer or book review site, I would appreciate it so much. It will encourage me to write more and it will encourage others to take a chance on my work.

I plan to add to the Relaxation Solution series. If you want to be notified of early-bird discounts, previews, and exclusives on my advanced courses and other materials, you can sign up here: **r.elax.in/news**.

I'd also love to hear from you directly. If you have a question or a topic you'd like me to cover, you can email me at **stephen@stephendiamond.me**.

Thank you.

The Relaxation Solution Workbook and Journal

About the Author

Stephen Diamond has studied and practiced mindfulness, meditation, self-realization, and nonduality for 50 years. He founded More Than Mindful in 2015 and launched The Relaxation Solution program in 2022.

A former singer, software architect, and political candidate, Steve began teaching mindfulness in 2015. He has taught public and private classes, coached private clients, and presented at gatherings large and small. His guided meditations have been played nearly 30,000 times on the Insight Timer mobile app, where users have rated them 4.6 out of 5.

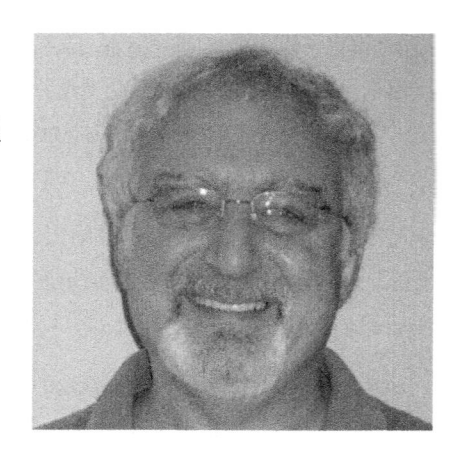

Steve is deeply familiar with various nonduality teachings, including Zen Buddhism and Advaita Vedanta. And he's practiced several types of meditation: TM (transcendental meditation), zazen, vipassana, metta, and mindfulness meditation.

In 2022 he brought all that experience plus new techniques and insights into his groundbreaking stress relief program, The Relaxation Solution.

Read more at Stephen Diamond's site: **r.elax.in/sdme**.

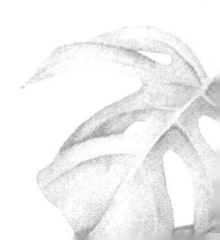

Made in the USA
Las Vegas, NV
12 January 2023